Plas Gwynant
Celebrating 60 Years

Sandra Meredith-Booty
& Frank Batchelor

Sandra Meredith Publishing

First Edition
Published by Sandra Meredith Publishing 2018

Book Design: Lisa Simone Jones

Paperback ISBN 978-0-9571279-4-4

Printed and bound in Great Britain by TJ International Ltd, Padstow, Cornwall

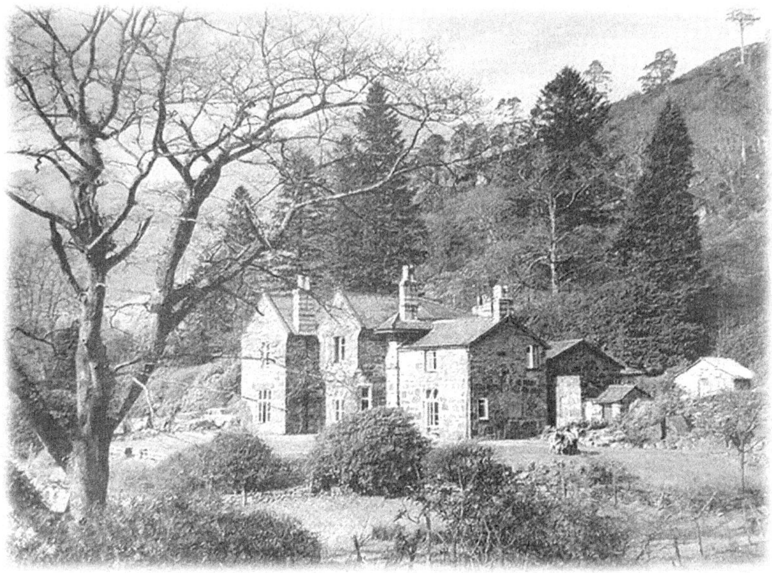

An Anthology of Memories Compiled by
Sandra Meredith-Booty and Frank Batchelor

The first course at Plas Gwynant was in May 1958, which paved the way initially for pupils of West Bromwich secondary schools, to experience outdoor activities in Snowdonia. Catchment expanded to encompass many more schools in the five surrounding towns when the council boundaries changed and became Sandwell Metropolitan Borough Council.

Sixty years later the expansion and improvement of the centre and the development of courses offered have continued to provide young people with possibly their first taste of outdoor pursuits and skills as well as a life changing love of adventure. It is hoped that the changes to education made by the far-sighted West Bromwich Council in the 1950s, recorded within this commemorative book, will become the legacy of their remarkable decision to purchase Plas Gwynant and their continued commitment to its success.

> *I do not need to emphasise the fact that not only are we not an educational 'frill' but in the present climate of unemployment, financial hardship and social disruption, when school children are questioning the value of the traditional type of schooling, the importance and relevance of the Plas Gwynant experience is increasing all the time.*
>
> Phil Watkin
> Former Plas Gwynant teacher

~ CONTENTS ~

~ PREFACE ~

When I boarded the coach on the morning of 16 May 1958 to go with a party of boys from Hill Top Secondary Modern School, West Bromwich, to camp at Plas Gwynant – the first party to go there, little did I know that some 59 years later that I would be asked to write a Preface to a book, commemorating the sixtieth anniversary.

In 1958 the house was not fit for use, so we camped. The weather was typical Welsh weather – it rained most days and we had to boil the spring water. As I wrote in the Camp Log, 'this proved a great handicap'. We were pioneers and Hill Top was always willing to give anything a go. Personally, it made me a firm believer in Outdoor Education. I carried this belief with me when I moved from teaching into the Education Office. Murray Watterson was a great Head and he set the pattern for those who followed him.

The Outdoor Education experience is something you always remember. Learning to work with others as a team is an experience that can be taken from school life into the wider world, wherever one goes after full time education is finished. Modern life is so individualistic, but when one is climbing Snowdon by one of the many paths, teamwork is so important – the strong can help the weak. Reading the journal, I noticed that the day ended with prayers; how life has changed over the years. I am sure that everyone will enjoy reading the history and be grateful for Ms Meredith for taking the time and trouble to research the archives to ensure that there is a lasting memorial to the farseeing individuals who bought Plas Gwynant and to those who have supported it ever since.

John Murden, Former Deputy Director of Education in Sandwell 1983

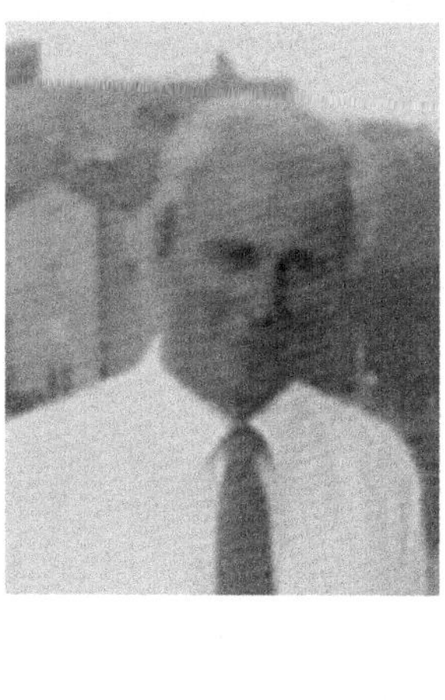

John Murden held a teaching post at Hill Top Secondary Modern School for Boys in the late 1950s and was proud to be part of the pilot course for its students. He later became Head of Department for Religious Education at West Bromwich Secondary Technical School for four years. In April 1963 he left to work in the Education Office, where he eventually became Deputy Director of Education for Sandwell in 1983. After retirement, John wrote 'A History of Smethwick Education 1922-1966' and 'A History of Warley Education Service'. He has also kindly contributed to this author's book 'The Cronehillians' in 2013.

~INTRODUCTION~

The Land of Eryri

Selected extracts from The New Naturalist: 'Snowdon: The National Park of North Wales' by F J North, Bruce Campbell and Richenda Scott, 1949.

In the detailed historical, geographic and geological study from the book 'Snowdon, The National Park of North Wales' it is easy to see how this rugged, untamed countryside challenged all who lived and worked in the area, transforming it into productive farmland, forests and unrivalled panoramic views enjoyed by thousands of visitors every year. In 1188 Giraldus Cambrensis (Gerald the Welshman) wrote:

> *I must not pass over in silence the mountains called by the Welsh Eryri, but by the English Snowdon or Mountains of Snow, which, gradually increasing from the land of the sons of Conan and extending themselves northwards near Deganwy, seem to rear their lofty summits even to the clouds when viewed from the opposite coast of Anglesey.*

The structure and perceived isolation gives Snowdon a characteristic pyramidal outline, recognisable from many viewpoints, appearing symmetrical. It is however, peppered with hollows with precipitous curving sides – the sharp ridges attractive to the climber, the striking views for the walker. The valleys separate tracts from the south east to the north west, but a fifth tract is isolated by a curved hollow that extends from Betws-y-Coed to Traeth Mawr and includes the valley of the Llugwy, Nant-y-gwryd, Nant Gwynant and the Glaslyn valley. But the most consistently beautiful of them is Nant Gwynant. It is in this area that some of the most important early attempts of reforestation were made in the nineteenth century by Daniel Vawdrey and others. The house named Plas Gwynant is situated on the south west facing slope of the Nant Gwynant valley and situated between the two ribbon lakes, Llyn Gwynant and Llyn Dinas, at a point where a tributary of Llyn Edno, passes to the front of the park. In 1803 the estate was sold by Sir Watkin Williams Wynn, to Daniel Vawdrey[2] Esq of Tushingham, Cheshire. The presence of this river with its waterfalls together with the outstanding view along the valley towards Llyn Dinas, Beddgelert and Moel Hebog in the distance, would have been significant in the choice of location, as well as the importance of the sheltering effect of the hills to the south and north. A description from 'Scenes in North Wales' by G N Wright 1833:

> *The vale here contracts, and the grand mountain masses rapidly close in forming the hollow of Cwm Llan, where Snowdon is observed to tower with greater majesty than in any other position. Beneath the darkening front and encompassed by a noble amphitheatre of mountains, is Plas Gwynant, the truly romantic seat of Mr Vawdrey. At this precise spot, the beauty of the scenery increases wonderfully, and the spectator is lost in an endless variety of rock, wood, flood and mountain, Llanberis Vale may be more sublime; no valley in Wales is equally beautiful.*

~HISTORY~

The Vawdrey Family

The Vawdrey family of Tushingham Hall and Ravenscroft Hall in Cheshire held estates since the Normans, Sir Claude de Vawdrey, received them as grants from Hugh Keviloc, Earl of Chester in the twelfth century. Daniel Vawdrey[2] (1771-1844) inherited the Estates and Halls at Moresbarrow and Tushingham, Cheshire in 1821, after the passing of his father (also Daniel Vawdrey[1], (1751-1821), who had previously gained inheritances via his maternal grandfather to considerable property from the Yates's of Middlewich (Dr Thomas Yate, Principal of Brasenose College, Oxford)

He was destined for the bar, and articled in the office of Messrs. Fox, Sharp and Eccles, Solicitors, Manchester; remaining for the customary period of five years, but succeeding to an independent fortune from his maternal grandfather did not complete his articles; (on the demise of his father he exchanged the role of a solicitor for the social retirement of the country gentleman).

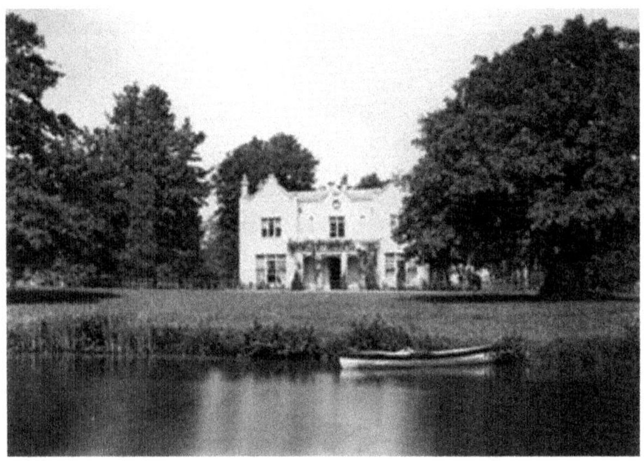

The grade II listed Tushingham Hall, park and ornamental lake was remodelled for Daniel Vawdrey who purchased it in 1814. It was originally an early moated farmhouse.

There are other names and associates of Daniel Vawdrey, the Wyatt family being the most significant. Daniel married Anne Wyatt (1783-1819) of Lime Grove, Llandegai, Caernarvonshire in 1804. They had three sons, Daniel Vawdrey[3] (1807-1896). William Seaman Vawdrey (1808-1877) and Benjamin Llewelyn Vawdrey (1809-1892).

Anne was the daughter of Benjamin Wyatt (1744-1818) who was chief agent for the Penrhyn estates and the brother of James Wyatt (1746-1813), an architect of national renown – Surveyor General to the Board of Works and Ordnance and considered a rival to Robert Adam in neo-classical design, and eclipsed him in his neo-gothic architecture.

The Wyatt's were a dynasty of architects and civil engineers of national and international prominence. Anne's brother also James, was to become chief agent for the Penrhyn estate on the demise of his father and played a prominent part in the development of the estates of Bryn Gwynant and Plas Gwynant. The estate was bought as a farm in 1803 and reported as being between 1000 to 1500 acres, the only residence at the time being the farmhouse of Hafod Anrheg (later Hafod Tan y Graig) some way up the Llynedno valley, and Glan Gwynant, described as 'a pretty little summer residence of the Vawdrey's at the south west of Llyn Gwynant'.

About the same time that Daniel Vawdrey[2] purchased the estate which would include Plas Gwynant, the adjoining estate at Bryn Gwynant, once known as Pen y Bryn, was purchased by a Mr Doulben, also from Sir Watkin Williams Wynn. Mr Doulben's descendents sold this estate to the Rev Hugh Wynne Jones Tre Iorwerth, in 1809, who used it to try out new farming methods, particularly forestry, believing this to be the way forward. Ideas which were in complete sympathy with those of Daniel Vawdrey[2]. Within four years of owning the estate, the Rev Jones had planted 160,000 trees, mainly Oak, Ash and Scotch Fir, laying the foundation of the woodland today. It was on this estate the earliest experiments in reclaiming waste land for valuable plantations were made.

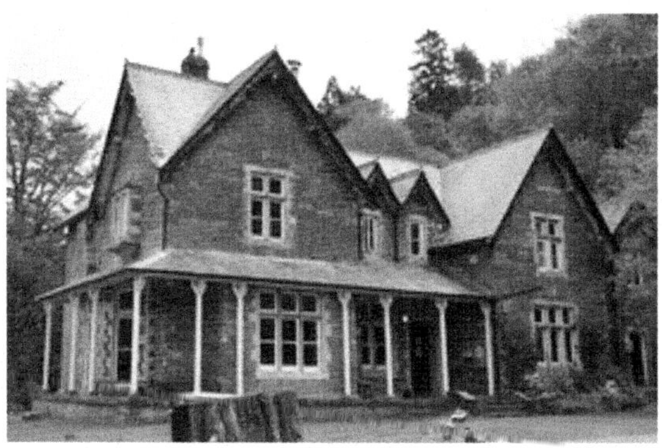

Bryn Gwynant

The house at Bryn Gwynant was built in 1834, shortly after the estate was acquired by the Wyatt and Vawdrey families. It appears that he and Benjamin Wyatt, Lord Penrhyn's agent, bought the estate. Benjamin was well known as an architect and was thought to have designed the house himself to use as a summer residence and described as 'typical of its period, being of dark stone with sharply pointed gables', today acquired by the Youth Hostel Association. At about the same time it is believed the current house at Plas Gwynant was remodelled and described as a dark stone, two storey house, unequally double fronted, with gables. The design of the two houses are similar, as was the style at the time, though in the case of Plas Gwynant, the two front fascias were an addition, leaving a distinct join between old and new brickwork.

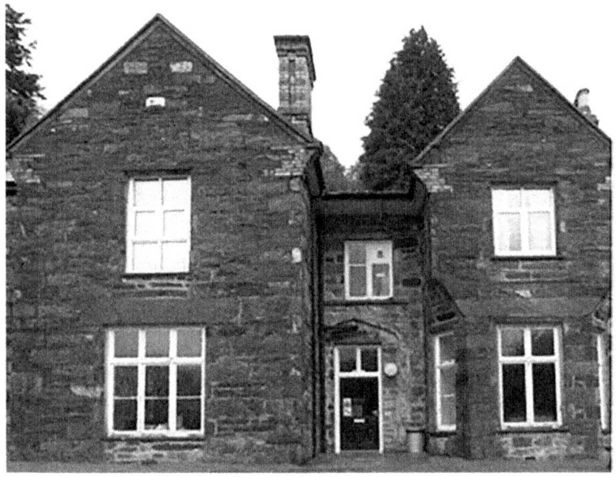

Plas Gwynant

Unfortunately, updating the frontage saw the ornate brick design around the doorway chopped off on the left side, leaving an interrupted arch around the entrance. Meanwhile Daniel Vawdrey[2] had also been busy planting 20,000 trees between 1808 and 1811. By 1818 the hill to the south west was wooded, the river valley to the south east planted and a plantation established on the south side of the higher hill, which has a picturesque walk and view point.

Further along the footpath there are constructed steps which lead to the base of Eagle Crag, where there is a natural rock 'table' which was enhanced with rock seats for family picnics. By 1824 there were ten cottages on the estate, two being the original farmhouses.

Daniel Vawdrey[2] threw his whole heart into the improvement of his property. He received a handsome silver cup from one society, and another for the planting of trees, from the Caernarvonshire Agricultural Society, where he later became a leading member. In 1829 he was appointed High Sheriff of Caernarvonshire by George IV (ref. the London Gazette 27 February 1829).

One account of his endeavours states:

> *The name Daniel Vawdrey, who bought the Plas Gwynant estate in 1803 is inseparably connected, not only with the travelling facilities which were introduced (the new road was laid through the vale in 1805), but also with the new energy which was breathed into the farming of the beginning of this century. He gave his tenants an example by tilling land which had never felt the plough, and turning apparently hopeless wilderness into splendid fields; and then created within them a spirit of competition by offering prizes to those who excelled in certain branches of farming.*

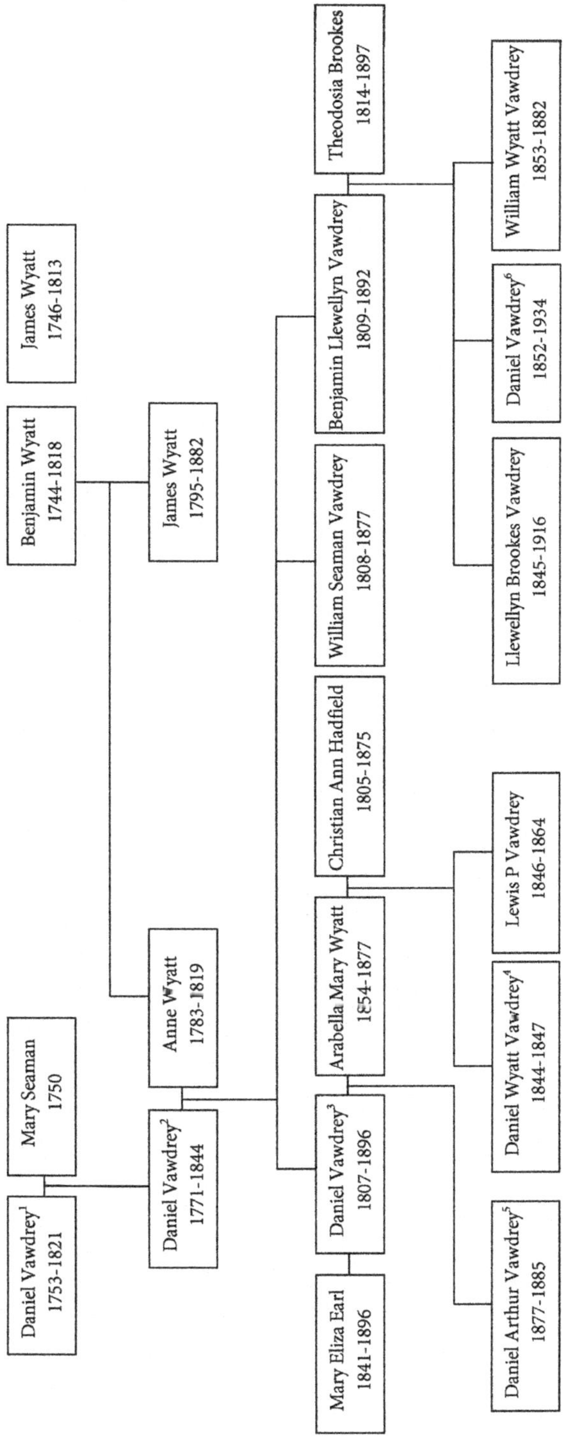

The Vawdrey Family of Tushingham Hall, Cheshire and Plas Gwynen, Caernarvon – linking into the Wyatt Family

Tenants and Notable Guests at Plas Gwynant

After the vale had been opened up by Thomas Telford's road between Shrewsbury and Menai, which was completed between 1820 and 1823, Plas Gwynant soon became a select spot. Almost everyone who saw it fell in love with it, and whenever it became vacant there was competition for it. None of the mentioned properties on the estate would have been the main residence of Daniel Vawdrey[2] and his family; as we have seen previously described as being 'summer residences' and so would have been let either to tenants or left to the care of the estate workers. There is however, evidence that Daniel Vawdrey[2] moved to Hafod Tan y Graig in 1836 (as referenced in featured ghost stories in 'Local Folklore').

The 1841 census has Daniel Vawdrey[2] (aged 69) and Anne (aged 59 registered at Hafod Tan y Graig, with three others (all agricultural labourers). Meanwhile at Plas Gwynant there is: Griffith William (aged 23), Miner in copper. His wife Elizabeth (aged 27) and daughters Anne (aged 1) and Mary (aged 3). On 14 January 1844 Daniel Vawdrey[2] passed away after only a few days illness in his 73rd year; a magistrate for the counties of Chester, Salop and Caernarvon. An extract of his will exhibits his desire to provide for the care of the estate after his death:

> *My son Benjamin Llewelyn Vawdrey is to care for my property especially the woodlands and trees. The woodland to be kept properly trimmed but shall leave as standards to grow into maturity in the proportions of one hundred trees to every statute acre of plantation and those to be left shall not be cut down or any of the ornamental trees at Tushingham, or Plas Gwynant within forty years of the date of this will, all my houses and buildings and goods to be kept insured from loss or damage by fire.*
>
> (Prerogative Court of Canterbury wills 1384-1858)

The estate passed to the Rev Daniel Vawdrey[3] (1807-1896) who was Rector of Darley in Derbyshire between at least 1851 and 1891 (UK Census Records). He had two sons by his first wife, Christian Ann Orford (nee Hadfield) (1805-1875); Daniel Wyatt Vawdrey[4] (1844-1847) and Lewis Pownall Vawdrey (1846-1864). Widowed in 1875, he remarried in 1876 to Arabella Mary Wyatt (1854-1877) and they had another son, Daniel Arthur Vawdrey[5] (1877-1885). His three sons predeceased him. His final marriage in 1883 was to Mary Eliza Earl (1841-1896). He was aged 75, she was 43.

The earliest mention of a tenant is a letter from a Mr J Coventry, asking for permission to shoot in the land at Hafod Ruffyd Uchaf:

> *1845 June 25, letter to J Hughes from J Coventry, Plas Gwynant. The late Mr Vawdrey had the privilege of shooting over Miss Parry's estate. He would like to procure the same privilege. What terms?* (Snowdonia Dendrochronology Project)

Apparently, Mr Coventry kept a good pack of otter hounds, which he left to the charge of William Jones, Castell. He was there for many years.

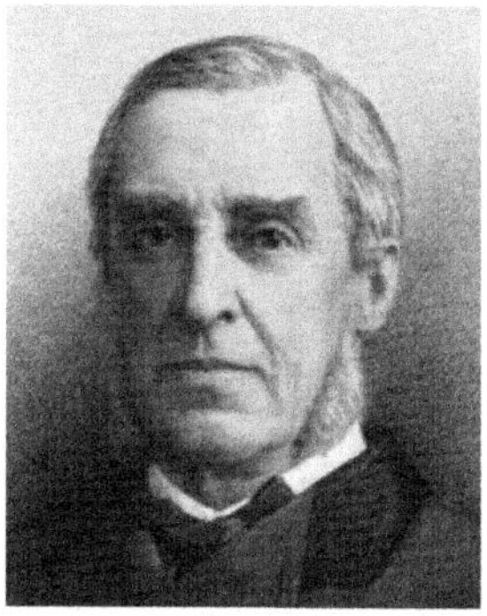

The Wales Census for 1851 shows the tenant of Plas Gwynant as James Anthony Froude (aged 33) of Dartington, Devon. His wife Charlotte Maria, nee Grenfell (aged 30) and daughter Georgina (aged 2 months). He took the tenancy in the summer of 1850 until the end of summer 1853. Whilst there, he wrote some of the best 'Short Stories on Great Subjects' and entertained many of his friends and colleagues. His published works include 'History of England: From the Fall of Wolsey to the Defeat of the Spanish Armada' 1856. 'The Knights Templar' 1886 and many more.

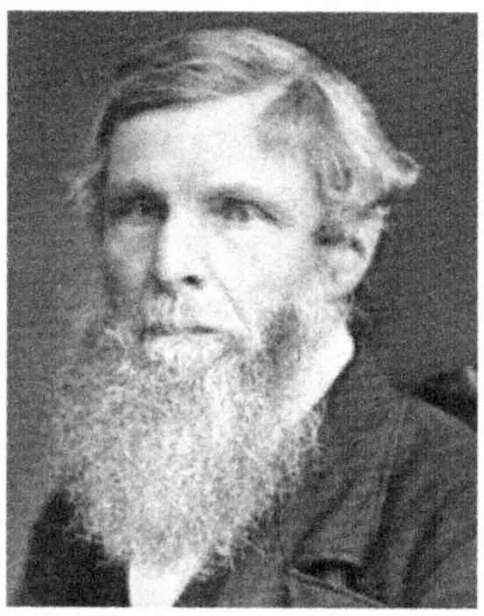

James Froude's equally famous brother was William Froude, who left the scientific world mathematical calculations that still ensures all ships at sea are safe. William was an engineer and naval architect who developed a method of studying scale models propelled through water and applying the information obtained to full sized ships. A similar technique was later used by pioneers in aerodynamics.

Several of Froude's college and literary friends visited him at Plas Gwynant and sometimes as many as six of the leading English literary men would meet there. Tom Hughes, Tom Taylor, Charles Kingsley, Francis William Newman and Froude himself may be just one of the several friendly groups that came together in those days.

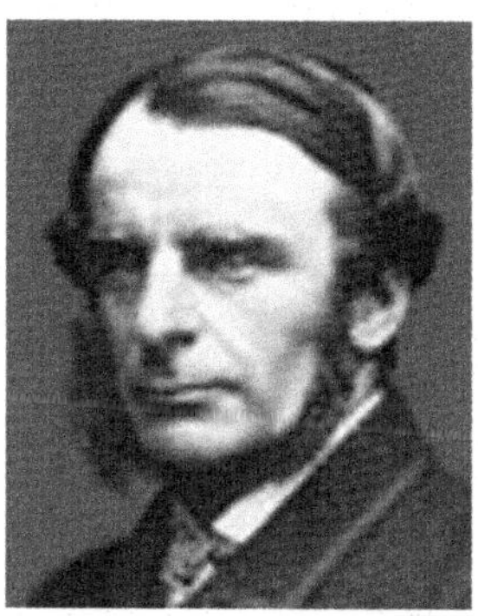

Charles Kingsley stayed at Plas Gwynant and undoubtedly enjoyed his stay there. Among his many books are 'Hypatia' 1853, 'Hereward the Wake' 1855, 'Westward Ho!' 1855 as well as his famous book 'The Water Babies'. It is thought that inspiration for the latter was during his stay at Plas Gwynant.

He also has the distinction of being among the famous who have fished at Llyn Edno, but legend has it that he had to be content with his picnic of hard boiled eggs and beer. His friend, author John Henry Cliffe however, in his book 'Angling in North Wales' in 1840, was more fortunate and caught six, averaging a pound each.

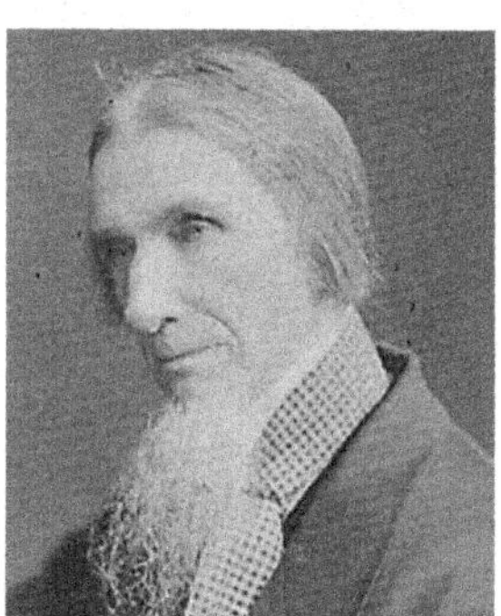

Francis William Newman, the younger brother of Cardinal Newman, was an English scholar and miscellaneous writer. Some titles from over forty books include, 'Phase of Faith' 1850, 'A Handbook of Modern Arabic' 1866, 'Iliad of Homer, Scholars Edition' and many more.

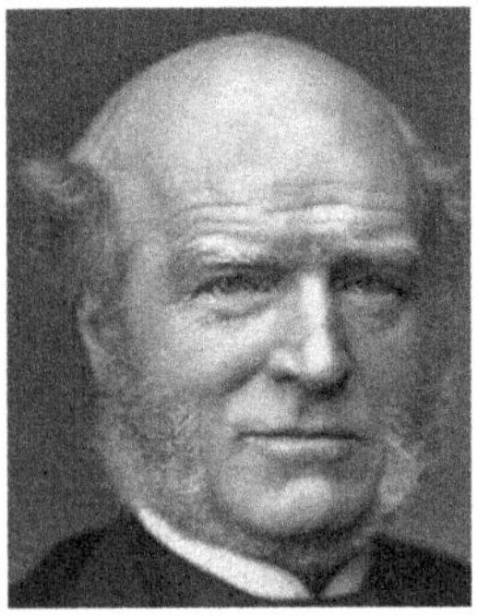

Thomas Hughes QC was an English lawyer, judge, politician and author. He is most famous for his novel 'Tom Brown's School Days' 1857: a semi-autobiographical work set at Rugby School, which Hughes once attended. He also wrote 'Scouring the White Horse' 1859, 'Tom Brown at Oxford' 1861 and many more.

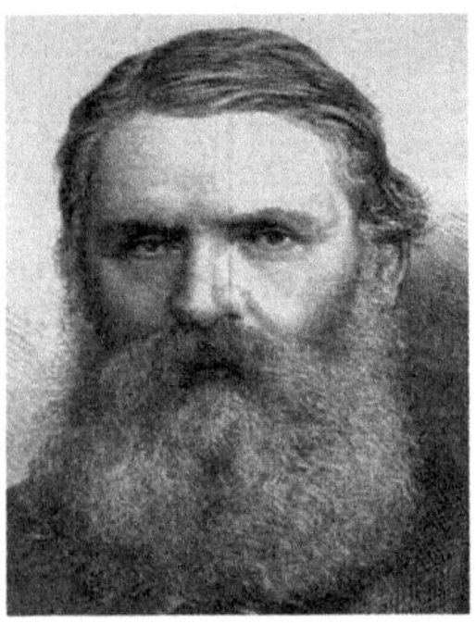

Tom Taylor was an English dramatist, critic, biographer, public servant and editor of Punch magazine. He wrote about a hundred plays during his career including 'Our American Cousin' 1858, famous for the play which was being performed in the presence of US President Abraham Lincoln, when he was assassinated in 1865.

Froude tried to get Plas Gwynant several times after he had left, but a lady called Miss Frances Minshall was in possession. Other occupiers gleaned from Census Returns are as follows:

1861 census - Frances Minshall, Head, Unmarried, (aged 58) Independent means, from Middlesex
Amelia Starke, Servant, Unmarried, (aged 30), Housekeeper, from Saxony, Germany.
Gwen Humpheys, Servant, Unmarried, (aged 23), Domestic servant, from Beddgelert

1871 census - Frances Minshall, Head, Unmarried, (aged 64), No rank/Profession, from Middlesex
Amelia Starke, Servant, Unmarried, (aged 38), Domestic/Housekeeper, from Saxony
Catherine Owens, Servant, Unmarried, (aged 18), Domestic/general, from Beddgelert

1891 census – Daniel Vawdrey[3], Head, M, (aged 84), Clerk in Holy Orders (Retired), from Cheshire
Mary E Vawdrey, Wife, Married, (aged48), from Yorkshire
Margaret Williams, Servant, Single, (aged 23), Domestic servant, from Beddgelert
Elizabeth Morgan, Servant, Widow, (aged 34), Cook, from Shropshire

In 1899 the tenancy was taken over by Miss Louisa Bannerman.

1901 census – Louisa Bannerman, Head, Single, (aged 57), Living on own means, from Eccles, Lancashire
Elizabeth Presnall, servant, Single, (aged 61), Housemaid, from Warwick, Coventry
Sarah J Jones, servant, Single, (aged 22), Cook, from Shropshire.
Florence Pritchard, servant, Single, (aged 18), Parlour Maid, from Radnor

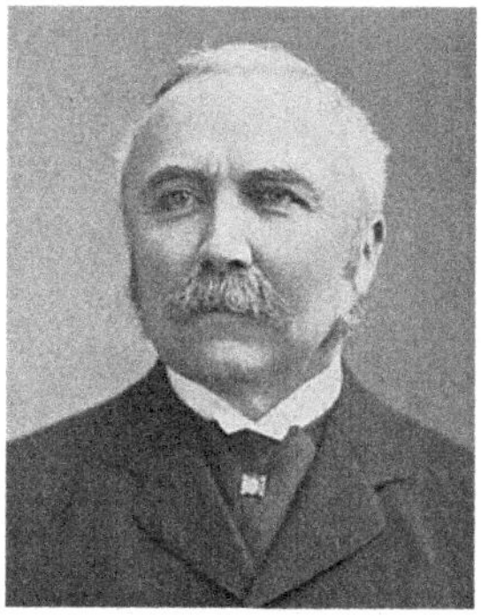

Sir Henry Campbell-Bannerman was a British Liberal Party politician who served as Prime Minister of the UK from 1905 to 1908 and leader of the Liberal Party from 1899 to 1908. He was the first 'First Lord of the Treasury' to be officially called Prime Minister, the term only coming into official usage five days after he took office. He also remains the only person to hold the positions of Prime Minister and Father of the House at the same time. It is highly likely that Sir Henry spent time with his spinster cousin Louisa Bannerman, who was a tenant at Plas Gwynant.

And finally, the latest Census Return available at present:

1911 census – Henry H Owen, Head, Married, (aged 51), Gardener, from Beddgelert Lazarus D Pereira, servant, Married, (aged 32), General servant, from India

On the wall adjacent to the equipment building at Plas Gwynant is a plaque dedicated to the memory of Henry Owen, long serving gardener at Plas. It reads:

'In memory of Henry Owen, for 50 years gardener at Plas Gwynant, who passed to his rest April 15th 1925. Delightful personality and a rare example of a happy Christianity and loyal service.'

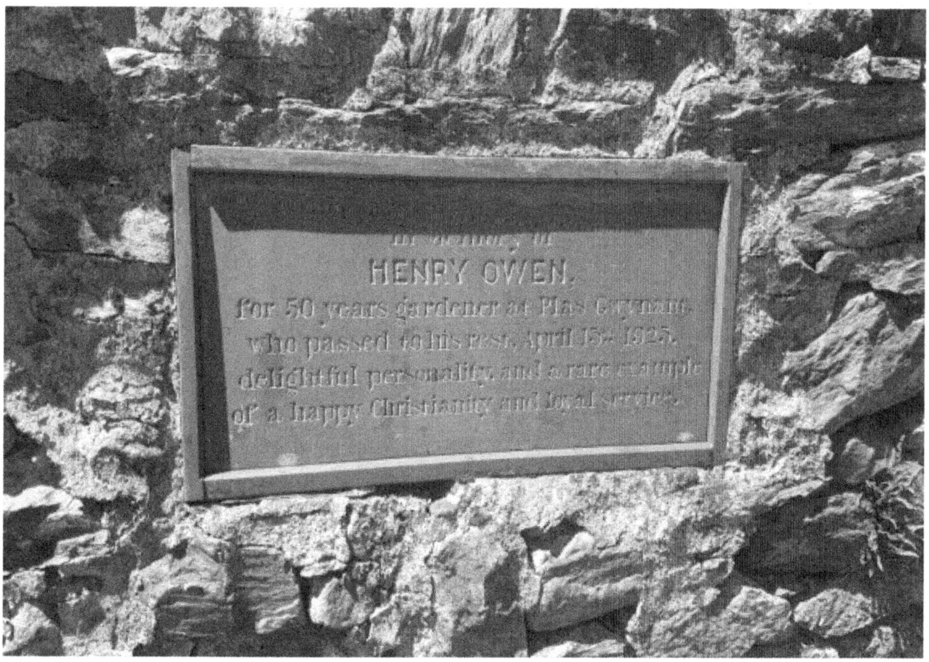

Roger Freeman and the Plas Gwynant Clock

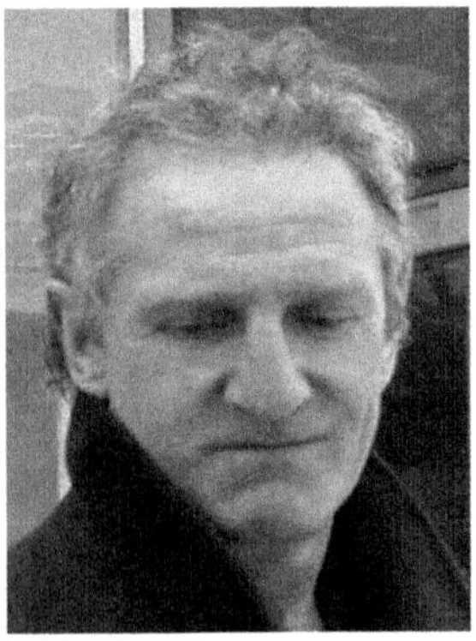

Roger (Paul) Freeman is in possession of the discarded clock with missing hands; thought to be well over a hundred years old. It still evokes a sense of history. Roger writes:

I found the clock lying on top of a dustbin at Plas Gwynant, waiting for the tip! I remember it from the time of the iconic and legendary Warden of Plas when we were there – George Simpkin. He idolised Rudyard Kipling and Lewis Caroll and used to quote them frequently – his dog was named 'Kipling'. All the clue-tins on our hiking treks contained phrases from 'The Jabberwocky' by Lewis Caroll. He also used to read ghost stories to us on dark and stormy nights to the hiss of Tilley lamps, (and we were in awe of him!)

I found the clock long after George Simpkins' time, when Murray Watterson was Warden and Plas was being extended. I doubt whether Simpkin, who was an arch-traditionalist would have ever thrown it out – it was the main timekeeper for the house and was wound diligently. It used to hang in the hall by the side of the stairs and got us all up and out onto the hills on dark mornings. The tale goes that it used to hang in the Plas Gwynant study when Charles Kingsley was a guest of the tenant, James Froude in the mid nineteenth century. It is thought that he was inspired to write 'The Water Babies' there. I was told that he got the idea from the stream and waterfall that runs behind the house.

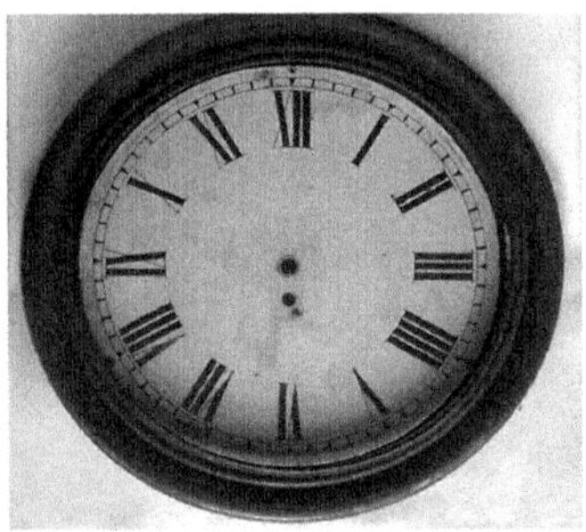
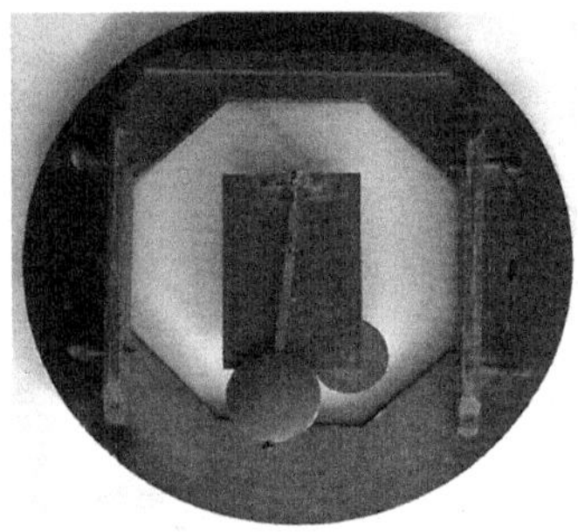

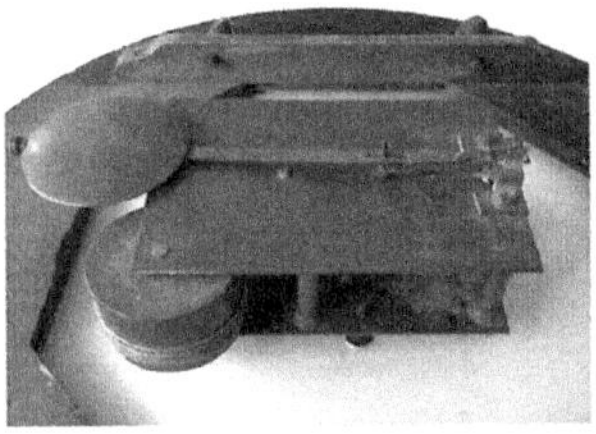
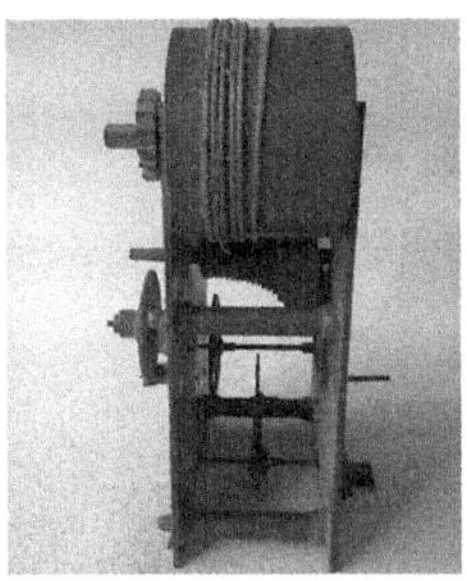
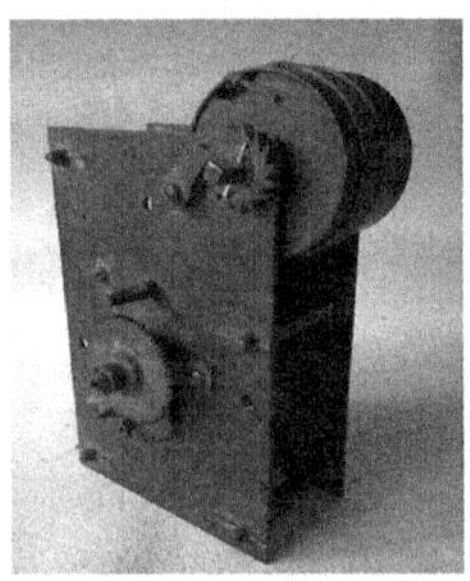
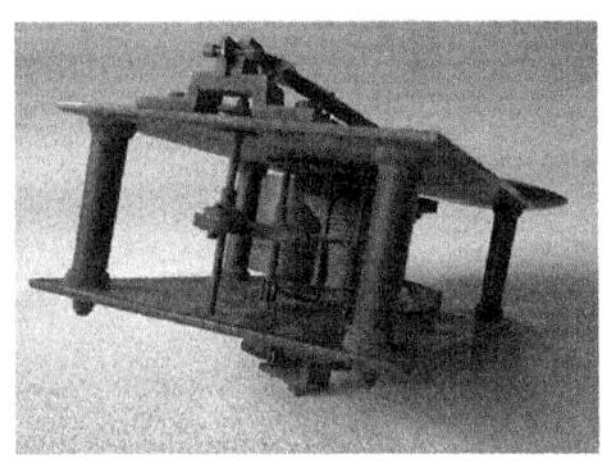

The clock itself is a 'Dial' or 'Drumhead' Fusee clock, probably made sometime between 1800 and 1880. The fact that the wood is oak as opposed to mahogany, means that it was most likely made in Wales.

The carved Oak Plaque above the Kitchen Hatch

The beautiful Plas Gwynant oak carving above the kitchen serving hatch, which reads: 'Better a meale of pottage With Love – than of fatte oxe with Evil Wyll'. It comes from Proverbs 15:17, which translated into modern English Bible means, 'Better a meal of vegetable where there is love, than a fattened calf with hatred. It is thought that this may have been an original feature of the house when improvements were made by Rev Daniel Vawdrey in the early nineteenth century.

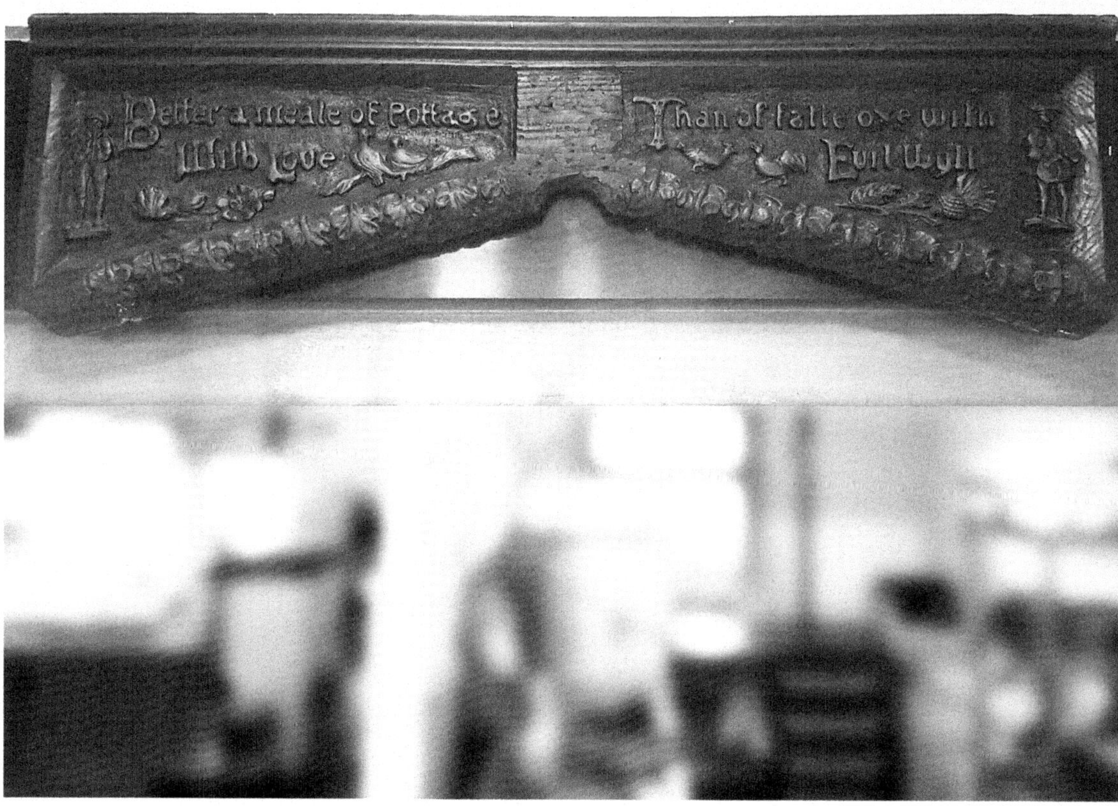

~LOCAL FOLKLORE~

Llyn Gwynant

From 'The Lakes of Eryri' by Geraint Roberts

The lake and indeed the whole valley was originally called Hwynan, Hwynen, Hoenen or Hwynwin (prefixed with the 'nant' in the case of the valley) whichever version certainly did not have the 't' which was added by the first owner and builder of Plas Gwynant, who wanted a touch of originality to the name. Many writers of some credibility including Sir John Rhys and even the Aberconwy Charter of 1198 testify the 't-less' version as being the genuine one. Gwynen may have been a long forgotten saint.

Plas Gwynant once had a troublesome ghost whose activities reached a peack in the 1840s. Unexplained noises and knocks were heard sometimes all night and whenever they were investigated the noises would occur elsewhere. The owner eventually offered free accommodation to his servants if they lived in. A newly married couple took up the offer and a trouble free period followed for two years. One night however, one of the other maids saw something that frightened her so much that is caused her to faint; she died a few months later without revealing the nature of what she saw. The ghost finally met its match in the form of Griffith ap Rhisiart who came to Plas to work and refused to be frightened. Quite soon it gave up its haunting altogether.

Another ghost that once troubled the farmhouse of Hafod Lwyfog for many months in the 1830s was eventually 'laid' at the bottom of the lake by an exorcist from Pwllheli. The ghost or goblin was a poltergeist that favoured nocturnal clog dances, knock over milk pails, lift and drop servants' beds and even squeezed somebody's leg so that he could not move for a fortnight. Another tale is told locally of two goblins that were caught roasting a young girl alive, one stormy night by her future husband. In trying to escape they fell over a cliff and were killed.

Yet another story concerns the disappearance of sheep, hens and food from various houses in the valley. One day an almost naked man covered in red hair was seen on the hillside by the shepherd of Bwlch Mwrchan. All attempts to capture him failed. Despite consultation with a wise man who advised them to pursue him with a red greyhound, the local farmers still failed to catch him, he would usually make his escape by leaping over a cliff. One Owalt, who stayed at home from chapel, heard a noise in the kitchen and upon investigating, she saw a red hairy arm coming through the window, she seized an axe and cut the hand off. The trail of blood was followed up the river Merch where it led to an inaccessible cave beneath the waterfall; the hairy man was never seen again.

Another version has the hairy man escaping over the mountain to take up residence in another cave by Clogwyn Du'r Arddu. Another fine old house which is near the bottom end of the lake is Bryn Gwynant. This was once called Penbryn and had the partial remains of what is thought to be a Roman paved path in the grounds. At one stage in its period it was a tavern called Pant Parlleni. Today it is a youth hostel.

The whole valley was once so heavily wooded that a man on a white horse could only be seen in one place on the opposite side. The spot is known as Goleugoed. The flat meadows at the upper end of the lake have for many years been a popular campsite and boating centre where hundreds come annually. The TV series 'Trailblazers' used the lake and crag on the north shore for a canoeing and abseiling competition in 1992. An old packhorse bridge crossing the river Glaslyn at the campsite is known as the Roman Bridge although it actually being Roman is highly unlikely. On the north bank of the river, halfway between the bridge and the lake is a well of clear, bubbling water and nearby a rock, which was used by an early Calvanistic Methodist preacher for open air preaching. Just above the bridge and old house by the name of Wenallt once stood, tradition has it that Madoc the discoverer of America stayed here during his preparations.

The last family to live here were startled one night by a huge boulder that had rolled down from the summit of Snowdon.

Ghost Stories from Plas Gwynant

Extracts from 'Bedd Gelert its Facts, Fairies and Folklore' 1899
By D E Jenkins, Porthmadog, Editor of 'Cyfres Ieunctid Cymru'

After the vale of Gwynen had been opened up by the new high road, Plas Gwynant soon became a select spot. Almost everyone who saw it fell in love with it and whenever it became vacant there was quite a competition among applicants for it. But at one point it took place rather frequently, as every occupant became nervous and restless after a few months. Something could be heard moving noisily over the house during the night, so that only the most indifferent could sleep in it. The frequent vacancies soon roused suspicion and the rumour spread that Plas Gwynant was haunted by a ghost. With the result that no one would take it at any price.

Mr Vawdrey[2] lived at Hafod Tan y Graig, or Glan Gwynant – it is uncertain which. He treated this ghost notion as an absurdity and determined to try and find out what was at the root of it. He got two bedrooms prepared one day and told his man that he wanted him to go with him that night to sleep at Plas Gwynant. After nightfall Mr Vawdrey retired to his room, leaving the servant in the kitchen. Ere long he could hear someone entering the house with a heavy tread and walking straight towards his room. He got up and opened the door, but saw nothing. He went to the kitchen thinking that the servant might have been in the front room; but he had not moved from his chair, nor had he heard someone walking heavily up the stairs and entering the room above his own.

He rang the bell for the servant and sent him up to see who was there. He found that particular chamber was locked, but could hear the sound of someone mounting the garret stairs and followed him. When he reached the garret everything was in perfect silence and order. While the servant was making his fruitless search in the garret, his master could hear some noise in the kitchen and had gone out see what it could possibly be. Both met outside the kitchen door, staring silently at each other in blank amazement.

The master was by now becoming a little serious, but did not yield his determination to spend the night there, and so told the servant that he must go with him to his room. As soon as the door closed behind them, there was a heavy knock on the outside, to which the servant attended. When opening the door, the candle was blown out so that the servant saw no one; the master however, distinctly heard the footsteps of two men entering the room. But after searching carefully every corner in it, he saw no one but the servant. In this way, both were kept going from one room to another until cock-crow, when stillness was restored and both fell off into a heavy sleep until morning. The following night when Mr Vawdrey was preparing to go again, the servant made the excuse that he was very ill and could not possibly go. His master was not sorry and never suggested the experiment again. In about eighteen months or so, one of the maids in Mr Vawdrey's service got married and he master offered her rooms free of rent if she wanted to live in and look after Plas Gwynant. Her husband was by no means a nervous man, and the offer was accepted. They lived there quite undisturbed for about two years, and seeing that nothing troubled them, they agreed to the suggestion of their master to pay a small rent. Almost immediately after the new arrangement was made, the disturbances began again, and the ghost became exceedingly troublesome so the young couple made up their minds to leave.

The evening before leaving, the woman was going out into the yard to fetch something and she was opening the door, some apparition appeared to her. On hearing her scream, her husband rushed to her and found her stretched out on the floor in a faint. When she regained consciousness she told her husband that she had seen something strange, but could not tell anybody what it was. She was never well again and in a few months she died, leaving the mystery unresolved.

After a time, a man by the name of Griffith ap Rhisiart entered Mr Vawdrey's service. He had heard the whole story about the ghost and offered to sleep in Plas Gwynant, if his master was willing. The offer was gladly accepted. Griffith was a religious man but retained his firm faith in ghosts, though he feared them not. He chose the 'ghost chamber' for his bedroom and before he had occupied it an hour, the ghost began to boisterously practice his antics. Griffith took absolutely no heed of its doings, until at last he became irritated and challenged the ghost to show its face and speak to him. He saw nothing, but the noise was increasing. It tramped the floors and stairs as if in wooden clogs, threw open the doors with a clash and dragged the bedclothes all over the room while Griffith was trying to sleep. All it got for its trouble was 'Well it matters not whether one sleeps on the floor or on his bed, as long as he does sleep!' At last the ghost got weary of trying to annoy this man and by degrees withdrew altogether. After Griffith's splendid, though almost effortless defeat of the ghost, tranquillity was restored.

A Mr Coventry, a gentleman of some wealth and position, took Plas Gwynant and made it the centre of a good deal of the sporting life of the district.

More Hauntings at Plas Gwynant in the 1850s

Extracts from 'Bedd Gelert Its Facts, Fairies & Folklore' 1899
By D E Jenkins, Porthmadoog, Editor of 'Cyfres Ieuenctid Cymru'

The haunting at Plas Gwynant seemed to be at an end and the house was taken over by a respectable sporting gentleman, Mr Coventry, who lived there for many years undisturbed.

In the 1850s it was lived in by the theologian and historian, James Anthony Froude who on many occasions enjoyed the company of his literary friends, Tom Hughes, Ton Taylor, Charles Kingsley, Francis William Newman to name but a few. On one occasion at Plas Gwynant get-together, Froude and his friends turned their conversation towards ghosts. Among other ghosts discussed, the one that had been troubling people in that house came under review. It so happened that Francis William Newman had only arrived that very day and the house was very full. Knowing that he was not a believer in ghosts or the possibility of their existence and hearing him gave such a free expression to his contempt for the notions which had kept alive the story of that ghost, Froude thought that he had found a capital opportunity on finding out how far Newman's ideas and beliefs protected his nerves. It so happened that the only vacant chamber in the house was Griffith's old bedroom, the 'haunted chamber'. Newman was put to sleep in that bedroom but was not told that it was haunted.

He appeared next morning after spending a sleepless night and made excuses that his journey had tired him out too much to sleep after it, while being in a strange bed came in for a share of the blame. He promised himself complete rest the second night but was disappointed, and for several nights he was continually disturbed. He then asked the housekeeper whether the ghost of which they spoke, sometimes disturbed the room in which he slept. She replied that it was the room in which it did most of its mischief, but that she had frequently slept in it and never heard a sound. He was greatly astonished, but gave none of the other friends any suspicion of his discomfort. At last things became insufferable and he told the whole story at the dinner table one evening. He said that he had hardly slept a consecutive hour since he had arrived, that he did not believe in the possibility of ghosts, but that something, but no means imaginary, was keeping up a continual disturbance in his room, and added that he wished to be excused the next morning; he wanted to return home. No amount of persuasion and offers of another bedroom could get him to remain. This happened during Froude's earliest months at Plas Gwynant, but the ghost never visited him again in Snowdonia. It was strange that none of Mr Froude's household either saw or heard anything of the kind during their stay, nor has anyone else since that time. Froude experienced no other disturbances during his tenancy.

Perhaps the spook moved on to Ewr.... ?

Ewr

Extracts from 'Bedd Gelert its Facts, Fairies and Folklore' 1899
By D E Jenkins, Porthmadog, Editor of Cyfres Ieuenctid of Cymru'

One of the most important stories in Beddgelert is the first hand account of an exorcism by a practicing ghost layer, whose name, disappointingly, is withheld. The exorcist described what happened when he struggled with a spirit at a farm called Ewr. Firstly, he explained that it was essential to determine the correct 'grade' of the ghost, so that you knew how to deal with it. Ignorance of the grade could prove fatal, he said. He told Jenkins that the Ewr ghost was 'an awful ghost, one of the worst I have ever heard of'. The way that he tackled it appears to tally with the technique employed by other exorcists, such as Griffiths of Denbighshire:

> *I at once consulted the oracles and after satisfying myself with regard to the ghost and its strength, I promised to go and put it down. One evening – I shall never forget it – I went thither and entered the house. I then made the mystical circle on the floor with salt and drew the image of the cross in its centre. Then I entered the circle myself and stood between the arms and the cross in the customary way, reading the usual charm passage. Almost instantly the door is flung back and some hideous creature, not unlike a huge tiger, enters, gnashing its terrible teeth at me. It then turned around the circle, as much to say 'I have it now'. I immediately perceived that I had mistaken its grade and that I had used too low a summons. But I stood like steel before him, showing not the slightest bit of fear and ordered him to withdraw in the name of the cross on which I stood, or else that I would curse him with endless torture. He stood unmoved and there we remained for a long time staring at one another, until at last I could see him gradually withdrawing. I then instantly changed one word in the charm passage and he came back, licking the floor like a dog before his master. I pronounced his sentence and sacrificed him to the bottom of Lyn Du; and while there is water in the lake he will never come forth to trouble anyone again. If I had betrayed the least bit of fear, or if I had taken my eye off for the quarter of a second, I would have been done for.*

There is no doubt that these accounts are indicative of the superstition that grew around all things not fully understood, or considered supernatural, especially in the nineteenth century.

However, myths and legends prevail in the collective memories of those living in the area – and who doesn't like a good ghost story?

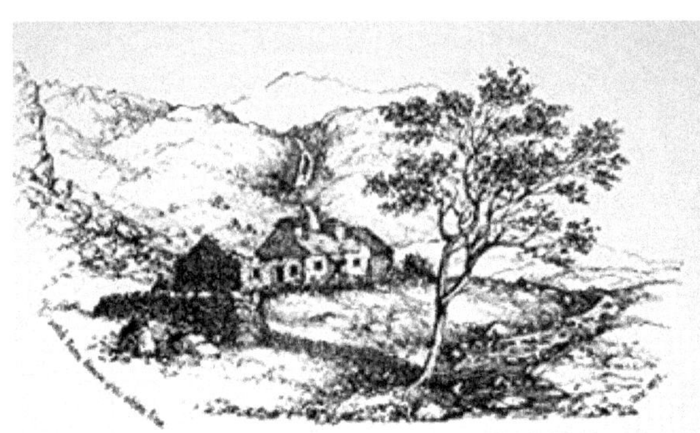

An 1873 lithograph by Daniel Vawdrey, featuring a farmhouse in Wales

Alfred Edmeades Bestall and Rupert the Bear

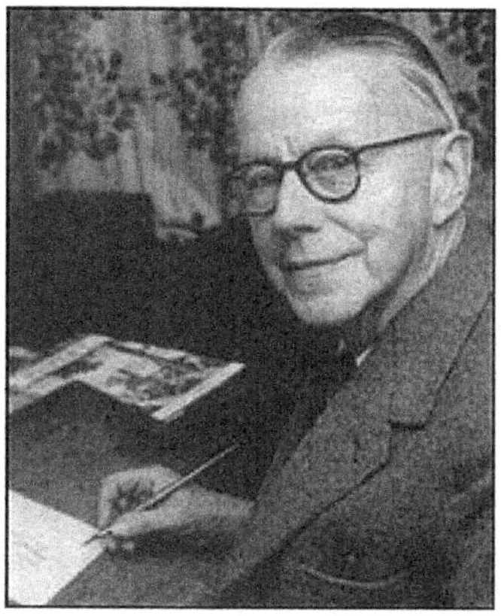

Beddgelert was the home of the late Alfred Edmeades Bestall, illustrator of the Rupert Bear comic strips and annuals.

Alfred illustrated the Rupert Bear stories in the Daily Express for 30 years. Invited to take over the Rupert Bear strip in 1935 when its originator, Mary Tourtel, had to retire due to failing eyesight, he developed and wrote over 270 Rupert adventures, and remained the regular artist and author until his official retirement in 1965.

He introduced new characters, Rupert Bear annuals, and ensured that Rupert and his friends always behaved correctly. Many illustrations resemble the Nant Gwynant valley, proving to be the inspiration for Bestall, who continued to contribute material up to 1982 and died in 1986 in Porthmadog. His close friend, Idris Evans also lived in Beddgelert and had many of Alfred's unpublished illustrations, all thought to be inspired by the Nant Gwynant Valley.

In particular, the three Sequoya trees opposite the Hut in the grounds of Plas Gwynant are recognisable in several of the landscape backgrounds in the Rupert storylines, though it is abundantly clear that the beautiful scenery in the entire area inspired Alfred's illustrations.

Idris was also friends with several members of the West Bromwich Mountaineering Club, who remember seeing many wonderful unpublished Rupert illustrations. Sadly, Idris died only a few years ago.

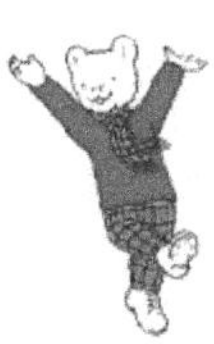

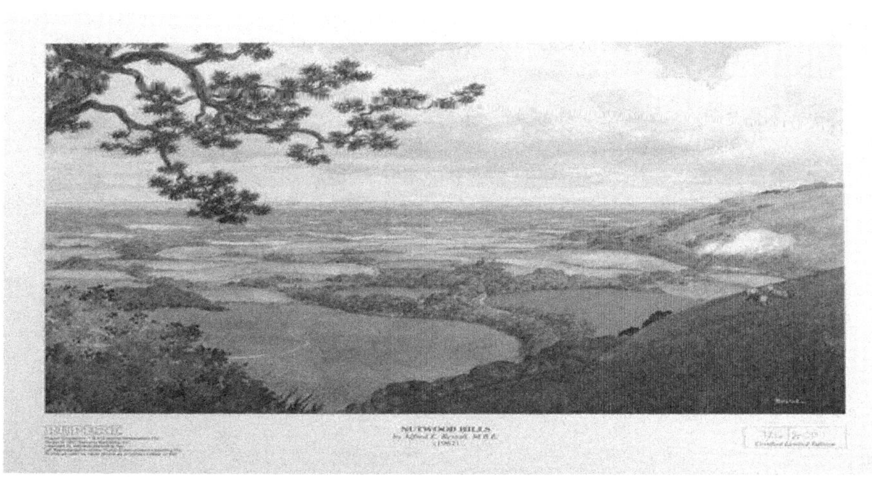

Nutwood Hills, from the 1962 Rupert Annual

~ WEST BROMWICH MOUNTAINEERING CLUB ~

The following contribution is an extract from their own book: 'West Bromwich Mountaineering Club: The first 50 years' by founder members.

The Club was founded by an enthusiastic group of teachers and friends, brought together by a series of innovative mountain leadership courses and schools' activity holidays during the post-war austerity years. Among the early members of the club were Bert Wright, an adviser to West Bromwich Education Authority; Geoff Robinson, Ted Hutton and Martin Bessell, teachers at West Bromwich Grammar School; Hughie Young, a teacher at Bratt Street School and Rev Keith Treacher of Lodge Road Unitarian Church. Other early members included Peter Woodward, Ray Vaughan, Mike Thompson, Wally Cheeseborough and Pat Tweedale.

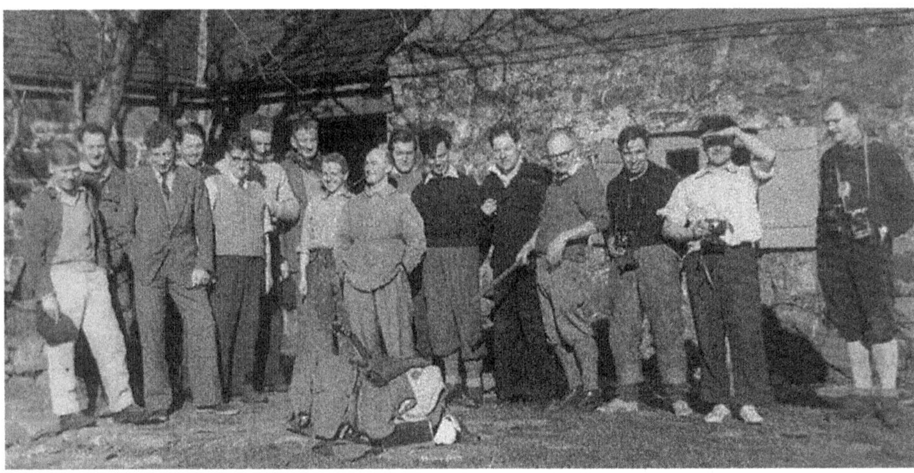

A Mountain Leadership Course at Helyg, circa 1958
Left to Right: Ray Mullet, Ray Highfield, Bert Wright, Hughie Young (glasses and tank top), A J Chester (Ches the cook), Pat Tweedale, Glyn Hughes (with pipe), Harold White, Ted Hutton (with stick), Pete Henk, Geoff Robinson and Brian Wilkes

When Bert Wright was appointed as an advisor to West Bromwich Education Authority in January 1951, he was asked to develop camping along with many other things. He found that one school had camped in the National Forest Park in Beddgelert, and being keen on mountains, he felt that this was a pearl that had to be nurtured! The number of schools camping grew and it was soon apparent that children and teachers were at risk because they were venturing into mountains with virtually no experience of the terrain and no knowledge of basic mountain techniques.

The obvious step was to arrange mountaineering courses for teachers. It was on one of these courses, probably through the misty haze of alcohol, that talk of forming a mountaineering club at either the Pen-y-Pass Hotel or the Pen-y-Gwryd Hotel – or both. But talking is not always followed by action; however in this case, there was an enthusiasm that carried through until today.

The club's first outing was to the Long Mynd in Shropshire in January 1952 and the club held its first meeting at the West Bromwich YMCA on 31st January in the same year. The next significant step for the club was the acquisition of a club hut in Snowdonia; a place of warmth and shelter that would be the base for mountaineering weekends nearby. A weekend away in Wales during the 1950s was not for the faint hearted. Arrangements were made as usual on a Thursday night in the Star & Garter in West Bromwich. The venue would either be Willie's at Ogwen or Farmer Watson's at Nant Gwynant. If rain was falling, it would be a quick pitch, stones under the top edge of the groundsheet and sides so the water would flow underneath. No sewn in groundsheets in those days! One would be lulled to sleep by the gurgle of water beneath you. Breakfast would be tea, tea-leaves in the porridge, porridge in the bacon sarnies and bacon fat on top of the second cup of tea. Then the serious talk about where was the climb going to be that day.

If the camp was to be at Watson's he would voice his usual moan about who had been washing in the stream and washing pans there too – it's coming through the taps! It was a different story when members took him to the Prince and plied him whiskey. Possibly one of the reasons he was happy to let them use the barn for their Hut! Farmer John Watson, who came from a long line of Farmers who worked the land around Plas Gwynant, was keeper of said hut and had a tractor which needed repair. As it happened, Bert was a dab hand at breaking and mending things and so had a go at fixing the problem. Luckily, it worked! It was a time when founder members were currying favour with John in the hope that he would relinquish the barn so that they could convert it for their use. It appeared to have worked, and a short time later the Hut was acquired for West Bromwich Mountaineering Club members. Then the hard work began to make it habitable!

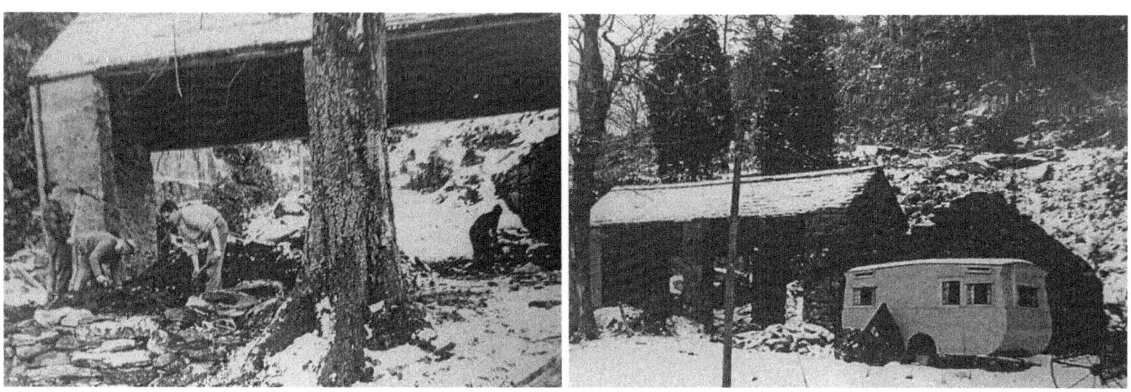

The Hut, used by West Bromwich Mountaineering Club, is situated halfway along the driveway towards Plas Gwynant House.

The positive endorsement West Bromwich Mountaineering Club received from Sir Chris Bonington CBE, was the Foreword for their published book 'West Bromwich Mountaineering Club – The First 50 years' co-written by the founder members of the club.

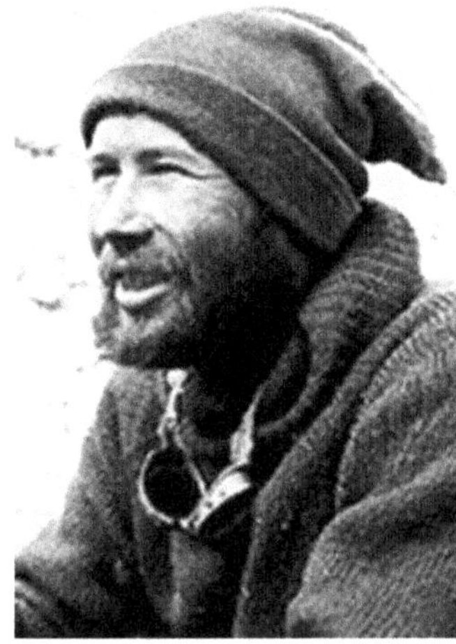

Fifty years is a long time in the life of any club. Just lasting that long is an achievement. Why has an average club like the WBMC thrived for fifty years? A common mountaineering interest among the members is one reason of course. Equally important, I feel, was the vision and determination of the small group of people who, in 1951, founded the club.

In spite of post-war restrictions, lack of transport, money and equipment, the club was born. Regular coach meets enabled members to get to the hills and by 1964 the club had its own hut in Snowdonia, thanks to the continued dedication of the early members. A camaraderie and sense of belonging developed and still survives. Hopefully it will help the club through the next fifty years.

With the membership of over 250, the club is active in the UK and many other mountainous areas of the world.

An average club? I think not. Its history and traditions have made it special to many members.

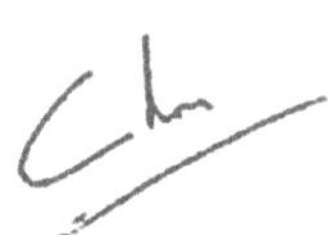

Sir Chris Bonington CBE
April 2002

The early links between the West Bromwich Education Authority (later Sandwell) cannot be underestimated. In fact, it is difficult to draw a line between the Authority's Physical Education Department and the early years of West Bromwich Mountaineering Club, so close was the link.

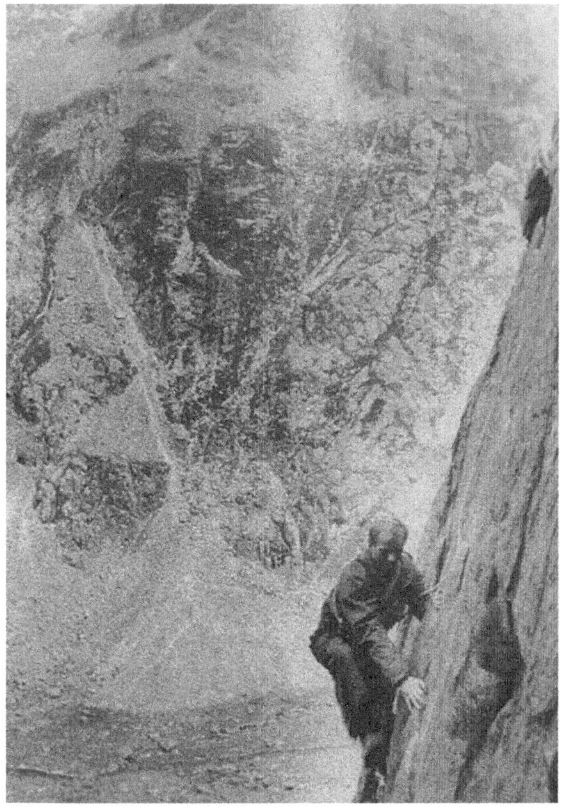

The legendary Pat Tweedale climbing Flaked Traverse on Dinas Bach, Llanberis Pass 1957

Nowadays the West Bromwich Mountaineering Club is run by, and for, mountaineers based in the West Midlands and surrounding areas. They have a diverse membership of well over 200 people ranging from children to retirees who take part in a wide variety of mountaineering activities, including mountaineering, rock climbing, hill walking and camping. They welcome complete beginners and experienced mountaineers alike.

The WBMC organise a wide range of mountaineering meets throughout the year. These include single day 'Coach Meets' to Mountaineering in areas in England and Wales and longer trips to these areas and further afield. They also run a wide range of social events, including dinner meets, evening walks and mountaineering slide shows.

After acquiring the Hut, interest was now directed towards the unoccupied house further along the driveway, which was now on the market – Plas Gwynant.

~WEST BROMWICH CORPORATION AND PLAS GWYNANT~

Why Plas Gwynant? Why did West Bromwich Local Education Authority end up purchasing a property in this beautiful, though remote, corner of North Wales? An article by Bert Wright may give an insight into the link with West Bromwich Mountaineering Club and West Bromwich Local Education Authority:

Bert Wright, Physical Education Advisor 1951-1976

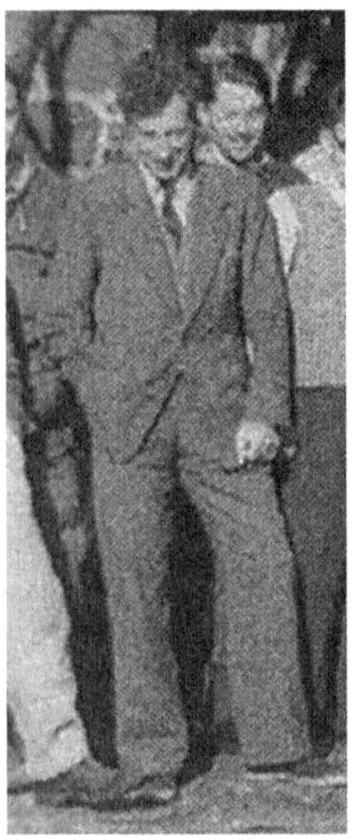

At the interview for the post of Organiser of Physical Education in 1950, one of the questions I was asked by Mr Turner, Director of Education in West Bromwich was "The Authority has a nebulous place called Shenstone Lodge near Lichfield; how do you think this large house could be used?" I well remember giving all the reasons I could think of why children from an industrial West Bromwich should camp in the grounds of Shenstone Lodge and use the facilities of the area such as rivers and Cannock Chase for canoeing and mobile camping etc. Incidentally Shenstone Lodge would not have been quite right for the job, would it?

A short time after I began working in West Bromwich, I discovered a piece of information which to me was like finding a tiny rare flower or a gold mine at the bottom of the garden. One school – Lyng – had camped in the National Forest Park, Beddgelert and had three or four ex US Army tents and a small garden party type marquee.

I had been introduced to camping and walking in the Welsh mountains when I was a scout and here I was working for an Education Authority which was prepared to spend money to extend the camping programme. Equipment suitable for the Beddgelert site was purchased and there began the gradual build-up of schools who wanted to camp. Without going into too many details this was not as easy as it seems now that I come to write about it. There were many factors that had to be considered before a school could camp. Some of these are relevant to this article.

a) Camping had to be for a period without any breaks. Schools had to be found who were prepared to camp in the Whitsuntide holidays.
b) Teachers had to have some basic knowledge of camp cooking, care of tents and other basic elements of camping.
c) Teachers had to have some basic knowledge of walking and safety in mountains.

I had to organise courses for teachers on site in North Wales and shorter sessions in West Bromwich. Gradually a 'hard core' of teachers who were excellent campers came together and gave great stability to the camping programme. Apart from camping, the mountaineering aspect had to be tackled. I had many friends who were mountaineers and I knew a little about it myself.

The result was many one-week courses at the Climbers Club Hut, Helyg, near Capel Curig, and one or two at Ynys Ettws near Llanberis. Gradually the camping programme became so much in demand that the 'season' often ran into the August holidays. In all these efforts, I was supported by Mr Turner, the Director of Education, who visited the camp and sometimes helped to dismantle the camp. The Councillors visited the camp and the Mayor and Mayoress paid an annual visit.

All of us who were involved with camping and our many visitors saw the value of children living and working together for a week. Schools placed their own emphasis on the activities they did in camp apart from essential camping duties. Some visited castles as part of a historical study, others visited the coastal areas, some walked in the mountains and very often the study was continued when they returned to school. The main weakness of the camping organisation was that there was no camp warden to foster good basic camping standards to look after the canoes, and to be advisor on safety in mountains etc.

We were very fortunate to get the Authority to agree to the appointment of a Camp Warden. This was a difficult job because three months living in a tent is fraught with all sorts of difficulties. However, the work done by Eric Amery and Pat Tweedale lifted the standards of camping and was an important link in the move towards a residential centre.

I travelled to North Wales many times in a camping season and it was about May 1956 that I saw the 'For Sale' notice at Plas Gwynant. How long it took to realise that 'this was the place' I cannot remember, but there was a further incentive to look at the property. In 1952 the West Bromwich Mountaineering Club was founded at one of the West Bromwich Authority's teachers' courses in mountaineering. A high priority for the club was a mountaineering hut and the Lodge at Plas Gwynant was one of the buildings we looked at. Plas Gwynant was not lived in and it was a short step towards finding a way to examine the property without attracting too much attention. On this first visit it was obvious that Plas Gwynant was the only place for an Adventure School for West Bromwich.

Many other exploratory visits were made during the camping season of 1956, but with nothing put in writing in the Education Office. However, Mr Turner had been kept informed and several Councillors were told about what was still only an idea. Councillors Fred Phillips and Philip Taylor showed a lot of enthusiasm. 1956 went by and the camping season of 1957 was soon with us and the 'For Sale' notice was still staring me in the face. Of course, the winter had not been wasted because in the West Bromwich Authority meetings between members of the Education Committee and those who worked in the office were frequent because the Committee room was in the office.

Opportunities to talk were many. Mr Turner favoured a centre in the Lake District, but during the spring of 1957 I was asked to present a detailed report on why the Authority should have a centre in a permanent building, as against working during the camping season from a temporary base. This report was completed and presented to the Education Committee with the knowledge that there was a property in North Wales which could be purchased at once.

In the meantime, an arrangement was made with the Outward Bound School at Ullswater for the Director, two Councillors and me to pay a weekend visit. As a social occasion, the weekend was a great success, and one of our Councillors was taken down a cliff face on a mountain stretcher, and two important points were discussed. Firstly, a lot of people we talked with thought that there were two Outward Bound Schools in the Lake District and that was probably enough. This placed Plas Gwynant into the number one position for future consideration.

Secondly, the Director offered my services as an Instructor for December 1957 at Ullswater where they were having their first course for Secondary Modern boys. I learned a lot in the thirty days at Ullswater which was to prove invaluable at our own centre. And while I was there, Plas Gwynant was bought by the Authority. The next phase was to get Plas Gwynant into use as an Adventure Centre. This is another fascinating story.

Council Minutes

The first tentative steps made by West Bromwich Council towards acquiring an outdoor education school were small indeed. However, the minutes from the General Purposes Committee Report, dated 3 December 1957, the agenda item 'Post School Leaving Course; Acquisition of premises at Nant Gwynant, Near Beddgelert' agree the go-ahead to purchase Plas Gwynant, as transcribed below:

<u>Post School Leaving Course – Acquisition of Premises</u>
<u>At Nant Gwynant, near Beddgelert</u>

> A visit was made to the Ministry by the Director of Education to discuss the possibility of acquiring a suitable property in the Beddgelert area for the establishment of post school leaving and other courses. A letter has since been received from the Minister stating that if the property could be purchased for £4000 and the minimum adaptations necessary could be carried out immediately for a few hundred pounds, the minister would almost certainly give approval to the project.
>
> Your committee had previously considered proposals for the establishment of a post school leaving centre and approval was given to securing if necessary an option to purchase the premises pending the authority to substantive proposals for the establishment of such courses. In order that the Education Committee could be in a position to move quickly should a sale of the Nant Gwynant property become imminent, approval was given to a recommendation that the Town Clerk be authorised to purchase an option if necessary.
>
> Since then, the Town Clerk has been informed that the Agents would be prepared to receive an offer for Plas Gwynant and the final negotiations will of course be subject to approval by the District Valuer.

Your Committee have considered very detailed reports of the Education Committee and the Borough Surveyor as to the state of the property and its accommodation and as to the cost of running both a pilot and full scheme.

The property when acquired would be used for the following purposes:

a) The establishment of courses of the Outward Bound type for young workers.
b) Similar courses for older Secondary School pupils
c) Nature Study and Geography Courses for Secondary Schools
d) The replacement of the existing Camping Site at Beddgelert

It is suggested that it would be unwise to run a full scheme in the first year. The existing camp will be transferred from Beddgelert and a number of pilot courses will be organised, using as far as possible, existing experienced teaching staff except for the Cook, who will be employed on a temporary basis. The Pilot Courses could consist of two of the Outward Bound type and two for Field Studies, and the enthusiasm of the teachers for this project is such that a volunteer force could be recruited to act as instructors for the initial courses and to carry out initial decorations and repair under the PE Organiser. In the light of experience gained in these Pilot Courses the scheme would be expanded so that the property would be in continuous use for 40 weeks for Courses of two or four weeks' duration. Assuming that the Pilot Scheme is operated next year, the total expenditure would be £892. The savings from the transfer of existing courses (£228) and the income from pupils (£240) would be £469 so that the total cost of the Pilot Scheme would be £424. As a first step in the development, therefore, and in order to meet the Minister's wishes, adaptations will be confined to providing adequate lavatory accommodation, hot water and occasional repairs. Eventually some consideration will need to be given to improvements in the living quarters as it is anticipated that some of the staff engaged will be in residence throughout the greater part of the year. Nevertheless, the standard of this accommodation need not be unduly high as the type of persons applying for employment of this kind would understand that the standard of living accommodation would to some extent be determined by the nature of the courses to be provided and the objectives they seek to achieve. The Borough Treasurer reported that whilst the revenue expenditure in the first year when only Pilot Courses would be held would be relatively small, the cost would increase substantially once the scheme was fully launched and detailed figures of estimated expenditure were submitted.

Based on these figures the net annual cost of the scheme when in full operation could reasonably be said to be in the region of £5500 to £6000, being £137 to £150 per week on a 40 weeks' course basis. The Finance Committee when considering the proposal did not approve it on the grounds that they did not agree as a matter of principle to the purchase and conversion of comparatively old property for this purpose and that on the estimate before them they felt they were not prepared to support a Pilot Scheme at a reduced figure.

Having considered all these reports and in view of all the circumstances your committee believe that the project should proceed and it is therefore recommended:

a) That approval be given to the purchase of the property, Plas Gwynant, at a price to be agreed by the District Valuer
b) That initial repairs and adaptations not exceeding £425 be executed
c) That the Town Clerk be authorised to complete any necessary agreements and that the Corporate Common Seal be affixed thereto as required, and
d) That accuracy be given for application to be made to the Minister for sanction to the borrowing of a sum not exceeding £4925 to cover the cost of this scheme.

Newspaper Article

Naturally there was interest from the local press and the Midland Chronicle Newspaper front page article dated Friday 6 December 1957, outlines the planned courses to be offered at Plas Gwynant, as discussed in the meeting and mirroring the contents of the minutes, the article has been transcribed here:

> West Bromwich Council at its monthly meeting on Wednesday decided to spend about £5000 on the purchase and adaptation of a property in Wales as a post school leaving centre – described by Councillor R T Spooner, (Chairman of the Education Committee) as a 'pioneering venture which, if it is a success, will probably be imitated by the country as a whole'. The property at Nant Gwynant near Beddgelert would be used for the establishment of courses of the 'Outward Bound' type for young workers; similar courses for older secondary school pupils; nature studies and geography courses for secondary schools and the replacement of the Corporation's existing camping site at Beddgelert, reported the General Purposes Committee.

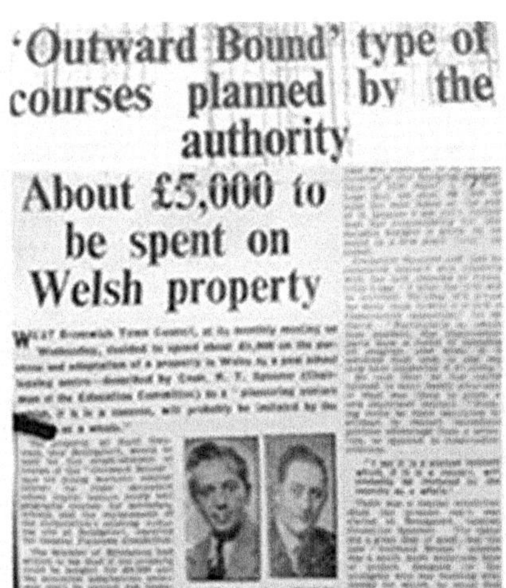
'Outward Bound' type of courses planned by the authority
About £5,000 to be spent on Welsh property

> The Minister for Education had written to say that if the property could be bought for £4000 and the minimum adaptations necessary could be carried out immediately for a few hundred pounds, he would 'almost certainly' give approval to the project. Negotiations would be subject to approval by the District Valuer, pointed out the General Purposes Committee report. It was suggested that it would be unwise to run a full scheme in the first year. The present camp would be transferred from Beddgelert and a number of pilot courses would be organised, using as far as possible, existing experienced teaching staff. Such courses could consist of two of the outward bound type, and two for field studies.

The enthusiasm of the teachers for the project was such that a volunteer force could be recruited to act as instructors for the initial courses and to carry out decorations and repairs under the PE organiser. In light of the experience gained in the pilot courses, the scheme would be expanded so that the property would be in continuous use for 40 weeks for courses of two or four weeks' duration, continued the report. Assuming that the pilot course was operated next year, the total expenditure would be £892. The savings from the transfer of existing courses £228, and the income from pupils (£240), would be £488 so that the total cost of the scheme would be £424. As a first step, adaptations would be confined to providing adequate lavatory accommodation, hot water and essential repairs. Eventually some consideration would have to be given to improvements in the living quarters because it was anticipated that some of the staff would live there throughout the greater part of the year. The Borough Treasurer had reported that whilst the revenue expenditure in the first year when only pilot courses would be held, would be relatively small, the cost would increase substantially once the scheme was fully launched. The net annual cost when in full operation could reasonably be said to be in the region of £5500 to £6000 being £137 to £130 a week on a 40 weeks course basis.

The Finance Committee when considering the proposal did not approve it, on the grounds that they did not agree as a matter of principle to the purchase and conversion of a comparatively old property for this purpose and on that estimate before them they felt that the eventual expenditure on the project would be too great, and that they were not prepared to support a pilot scheme at the reduced figure, stated the General Purposes Committee Report.

The Council decided, on the recommendation of the General Purposes Committee, to approve the purchase of the property at a price to be agreed by the District Valuer; that initial repairs and adaptations not exceeding £425 should be carried out and that authority should be given for application to the Minister for sanction to the borrowing of a sum not exceeding £4926 to cover the cost of the scheme.

Councillor R M Wimbury (Cons) commented that £5000 was only an initial expenditure. At a time when they were talking a lot about curtailing their expenditure, they were asked to pass expenditure of £5000 on a house that he had not seen but had heard was in a very bad state of repair. "We can see this immediately because we are told that the house had no lighting facilities and that the sanitary arrangement is very poor indeed. It seems rather ludicrous to me when only a month ago the Council decided they could not afford to spend £200 - £300 on toilets, which were badly needed for teachers on the Lodge Estate School, that we should be asked to spend £5000 on a tumble-down house in Wales I feel certain that this amount of money could be spent much more wisely on 'other' educational fields and put to much better use." Councillor P H Lugg (Cons) spoke of the 'Education Committee's hunting, shooting, mountaineering and fishing lodge'. "What if we buy it and have it left on our hands" he asked, "I don't think we want this broken-down Welsh mansion on our hands, without electricity and gas and it only has a private drainage system, which I have no doubt was constructed for the use of one household, not to be turned into an education establishment, which would mean it would have to be

considerably increased at some expense. We heard on a previous occasion, and I think it is fair to comment on it, that the cost of running this establishment would be equivalent to a 3d rate each year. That statement was made by a member of the Finance Committee. He may prove to be right or wrong, but I feel it is a piece of knowledge the public ought to have".
Councillor Lugg said that he thought that the idea of a post school leaving course was a good one, but thought that the proposed scheme was likely to be very expensive. "I appeal to you to throw it out on expense alone" he declared. "There was an alternative – the present Beddgelert camp. I hope the Socialist members on the Council who have objected to and oppose this scheme up to the present time, will continue to do so and because of the financial implications of this report, I for one hope that we shall be able to have the vote taken at the end of it because I am quite certain that the responsibility for this decision tonight is going to be noted in a few years' time" he ended.

Councillor Spooner (Lab) stated that he associated himself sincerely with the last remarks of Councillor Lugg. "I hope the vote will be recorded. Nothing will please me more than having a record of Conservative opposition" he declared, "particularly in education matters, the Conservative party have a habit of opposing all progress, and when it is achieved, they cash in and say they have supported it all along." He said that he had rarely listened to more feeble criticism of what was likely to prove a very important venture. "Nothing could be more calculated to attempt to extract immediate political advantage as opposed to constructive criticism. I say it is a pioneer venture, which, if it was a success will probably be imitated by the country as a whole."

"There was similar scepticism when the present camp was started in Beddgelert", recalled Councillor Spooner. "The camp did a great deal of good – but the new 'Outward Bound' scheme was a much more ambitious type of project designed for the youngster who was bursting with energy for which he could find no normal outlet in West Bromwich. Sometimes that energy finds an unfortunate outlet in smashing up a public lavatory, desecrating a public garden or hacking at trees. Part of the educational problem of the borough is to harness this energy and turn it into the right channels and the type of course given at the Outward Bound centre would open up a field of endeavour and interest which could last much longer and might affect the youngster for life." "Councillor Wimbury, in a very misjudged speech for someone who acknowledged that he had not seen the place, implied that they were buying a tumble-down ruin", continued Councillor Spooner, "we shall buy it at the District Valuer's valuation or below it and if he is going to value a tumble-down ruin at £4000 odd I am astonished, they are most careful at assessment of properties particularly those bought by local corporations", commented Councillor Spooner. "There was no electricity in the valley. If there was, they could not buy the property for anything like the price they were going to have it for. We are not going to produce what Councillor Lugg implied – something in the nature of a luxury hotel.

In fact, the essence of these courses is that boys and girls taking part will be as much as possible, self-sufficient", he stressed. "The other implication in the talk of a 3d rate was that in the long run it was going to be a very lavish and expensive scheme.

It would be money well spent stressed Councillor Spooner. "It would only cost a lot if the thing was an overwhelming success". He felt confident that in the years to come the people of West Bromwich would congratulate the Education Committee on their initiative.

Councillor G Hawkins (Cons) emphasised that they had no opposition to the proposed courses in principle. The opposition was purely and simply to the purchase of a property which they thought was a very bad investment.

(.........Sixty years later!)

More Council Minutes

A further report is provided to the Committee on 5 March 1958 under the agenda item 'Equipment for Plas Gwynant and is transcribed here:

Equipment for Plas Gwynant

Your Committee recommend that the following items of equipment, amounting to £603. 11s. 7d for which provision has been made in the current year's estimates, be purchased for the camp site attached to Plas Gwynant.

A.	From City Camp and Sports (1953) Ltd., 86-87 Broad Street, Birmingham 15		
	4	Torches in rubber case @ 7s. 3d	£1. 9s. 0d.
	3	100' x 1¼" Nylon Ropes @ 99/- less 10%	£13. 7s. 4d.
	3	120' x 1¼" Nylon Ropes @ 118/- less 10%	£15. 18s. 7d.
	10	Abseil slings @ 9/6d. less 10%	£4. 5s. 9d.
	10	Stubai-screw fastenings @ 12/6d. less 10%	£4. 13s. 9d.
	21	Standard Model Anoraks @ £3. 16s. 6d. less 25%	£60. 4s. 11d.
	21	Icelandic Standard sleeping bags @ £7. 2s. less 25%	£111 16s. 6d.
	5	Polished Plated Tilley Lamps @ £4. 2s. less 15%	£17. 8s. 6d.
	10	Type '5' (Scout) Compasses @ 15/- less 15%	£6. 7s. 6d.
	25	'Solo' canteen pots @ 16/3d. less 25%	£15. 4s. 8d.
	25	Polythene mugs @ 2/8d. less 25%	£2. 10s. 0d.
	25	Aluminium plates 9" diameter @ 2/5d. less 33.1/3%	£2. 0s. 3d.
	25	Knife, fork and spoon sets @ 4/2d. less 33.1/3%	£3. 9s. 5d.
	12	'Ever-ready' hand torches @ 7s. 2d.	£4. 6s. 0d.
	25	'Baby' can openers @ 6d.	12s. 6d.
	25	Water-proof match boxes @ 6d. less 25%	9s. 5d.
	24	Rucksacks – Super senior @ £6. 6s. less 15%	£128. 10s. 5d.
B.	Benjamin Edgington & Sons, Shaftesbury Avenue, London		
	4	2-man tents @ £12 each	£48. 0s. 0d.
C.	From Vono, Tipton, Staffs		
	11	'Champion double tier tubular bunks 2' 6" x 6' 2" including 'Calypso' inner spring mattress @ £16. 9s.	£162. 17s. 1d.
			£603. 11s. 7d.

The Borough Treasurer has reported that the provision in the current rate estimates for Training Courses includes a specific amount of £600 for Outward Bound type courses. This sum is available to meet the proposed expenditure (603. 11s. 7d.) which will rank for Government Grant at the rate of 60%.
The Finance Committee have approved the proposal.

At another General Purpose Committee held on 4 February 1959, agenda item 'Development of Plas Gwynant Adventure School' is transcribed below:

Development of Plas Gwynant Adventure School

Because of the outstanding success of the Pilot Course organised at the Plas Gwynant Adventure School last year and the requests for information as to what developments are envisaged for 1959, the Education Committee are of the opinion that the full scheme of development should be undertaken this year. When your Committee considered this project, the Chairman of the Education Committee gave an undertaking that Pilot Schemes would be run for the first two years, but having regard to the demands now being made for an extension of the facilities there, your Committee recommend that approval be given to the full development of the Plas Gwynant Scheme one year earlier than was anticipated.

It is therefore recommended:

1) That the following additional equipment be purchased:

4	Beds York No.5 3ft and mattress for staff use @ £13. 11s. 4d.	£54. 5s. 4d.
52	Pairs of sheets 63" x 100" @ 35/- per pair	£91. 0s. 0d.
104	Blankets 70" x 90" unused RAF blue @ 23/6d each	£122. 4s. 0d.
24	Good Companions sleeping bags @ £2. 13s 6d.	£64. 4s. 0d.
26	Ice Axes @ £2. 8s. 10d.	£63. 9s. 8d.
4	Mountain tents complete @ £19. 0s. 7d.	£76. 2s. 4d.
4	Edgington two-man tents and ground sheets @ £15	£60. 0s. 0d.

Kitchen Equipment

All items for cooking and feeding	£91. 10s. 0d.

2) That the Borough Surveyor be authorised to undertake the following alterations to the promises:

a)	Drying Room	£200. 0s. 0d.
b)	Repair of second outside W.C.	£120. 0s. 0d.
c)	Alterations to existing Bathroom	£30. 0s. od.
d)	Provision of wash-basins for use by boys	£120. 0s. 0d.

The Borough Treasurer has reported that provision for the proposed expenditure has been made in the draft rate estimates for 1959/60. The Finance Committee approved the proposal.

A final Committee meeting held on 10 December 1959, agenda item 'Plas Gwynant Adventure School – Tenders for Food Supplies 1960/61' is transcribed below:

Plas Gwynant Adventure School - Tenders for Food Supplies 1960/1961

Your Committee recommend that tenders for Food Supplies to the Plas Gwynant Adventure School for the year 1960/61 be accepted as follows:

Supplier	Commodities	Conditions
William Jones	Groceries and General	Approved provisionally For 6 months in the first instant
Caernarvon Dairies Ltd Eryri Terrace, Caernarvon	Milk	ditto
Deudraeth Bakery Co. Penryheudrath	Bread	Full acceptance
Richard Newell Ltd Central Buildings, Porthmadog	Meat	Full acceptance

It is further recommended that in the absence of any tender for the supply of fruit and vegetables, the existing supplier Alma's be invited to continue for the year 1960/61, and that the Town Clerk be authorised to prepare, sign and seal any contracts which may be necessary.

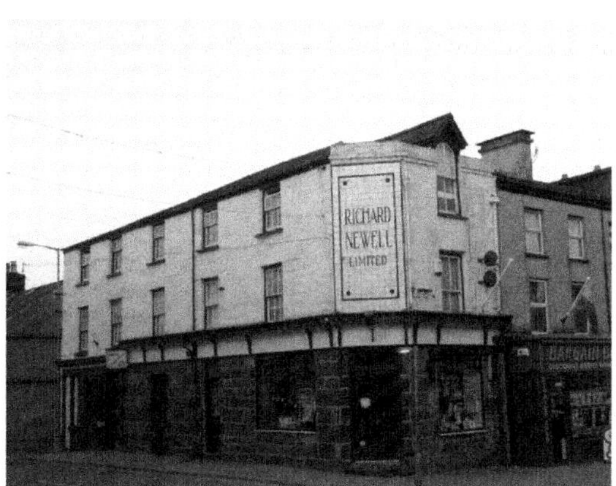

Richard Newell, Porthmadog

An extract from the pamphlet produced by Sandwell Department of Education 'Plas Gwynant The First 25 Years 1958-1983'.

J M (Murray) Watterson OBE

Head of Plas Gwynant and former teacher at Churchfields Comprehensive School

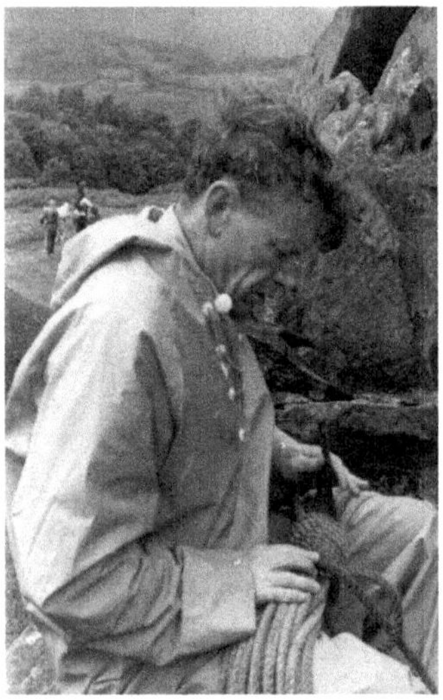

To buy the house was one thing, to open it as a centre was another matter entirely.

The situation of the house was magnificent. It could not have been better. The size of the house was very suitable and the size and arrangement of rooms proved to be more adaptable than anyone could have envisaged. Nevertheless, there was no electricity – none in the valley except for certain farms who generated their own via small hydro-electric schemes, and there was no comprehensive sewage disposal – it just went! (to where nobody ever really knew).

Although there was plenty of good quality available water, the storage of an amount needed to cope with the needs of twenty odd youngsters plus instructors, was totally inadequate. The latter situation presented no great problem. A 25,000-gallon concrete storage tank was constructed and except towards the end of the 1976 drought, this has provided all the water we need, and of the very highest quality.

The lack of electricity presented the greatest problem in running the Centre, although for course members at the time, it probably remains one of the outstanding memories of the place. Tilley lamps spluttering in the hall, dark 'spooky' corners (the boot room), refuelling and cleaning out the Aga cooker and solid fuel boiler. In fact, living in the very rudimentary world about which they had only read, and providing an added element to the 'adventure' soon became a frustration. Alright for those who only spent 26 days on the course, but often a misery for permanent staff, represented by the 14 lamps to be 'fettled up' at the beginning of the course rapidly dwindling to 8 which then had to remain in the hallway to be collected if anyone had to move from one part of the building to another; the ever-present smell of paraffin from ones clothes due to the fine jet directed up the arm as the pressure was released; the danger from the meths fires in the shed; the dirt in the kitchen from the refuelling of the fires with often damp fuel; the fumes from the water boiler; nothing was ever clean and every little job was a difficult chore. Roll on the electricity supply! But it must be admitted that there was something about those days, which even I, suffering all the frustrations, the fears of the risk of fire and the organising of the duty instructor to 'go back to Plas, light the Tilley's and the drying room fire' at 2 in the afternoon. I'm not sorry I experienced them all. The electricity duly arrived in 1966 and the progress of the poles advancing down the valley excited everyone. When the supply did not arrive in time for

Christmas, a little elderly neighbour was overheard to say, "Never mind, perhaps it will be here for next Christmas!" There's patience for you, fair play!

The arrival of the power really did provide tremendous relief – from fire (although the only serious fire the Centre has known was the result of an electrical fault!) and from the heavy chores of the daily grind. To have the convenience of a refrigerator, a drying room heated at the touch of a switch, vacuum cleaners to suck up instead of distribute dirt and above all, light, meant that more time could be spent on the hills, which is what the Centre is about. There is no doubt that the carrying out of necessary chores contributes in a major way to the success of a course, but there is a limit.

The year 1967 was a memorable year. Proper sewage disposal arrangements were built, the first extension to the building was planned and foot and mouth disease arrived. Travel through the badly infected areas of Shropshire was discouraged as was the use of the hills in case the disease spread across North Wales. Happily, it did not, and happily also, the resulting cancellation of courses provided the opportunity to press on with the modernising of the kitchen and the construction of a drying room with field study and games room. The building of more dormitory space was stopped by the first of the financial squeezes and did not finally materialise until 1974 with the creation of the new Borough of Sandwell, when the capacity of Plas Gwynant was finally increased to 40 places.

All those who were involved in the early courses will remember that they were 26 days in length. Originally this was because the Centre was intended to run along Outward Bound lines. The activities and methods of operation were similar in every respect. Eventually the length of the course was found to be not convenient for many reasons and it was reduced by 7 days. This course in turn was proved to be extremely popular so that demand far outstripped the places available. After consultation in which Her Majesty's Inspectors were also involved, it was decided that the course could be reduced by a further 7 days to its present length provided that the original principles could be applied and strictly adhered to. As a result, courses are shorter but more intensive and there is no doubt whatever that the loss in length of time is at least made up by the quality of the experience.

The title of the Centre was originally Plas Gwynant Adventure School. It was changed to Plas Gwynant Outdoor Education Centre at a time when the term 'Adventure' seemed to suggest unnecessary frills to education and so to call it an Outdoor Education Centre would suggest respectability. Perhaps it is a more accurate title since it now also offers academic courses in Field Studies and opportunities for teachers to train in Outdoor Activities. However, to me the main course will always constitute the 'Adventure School' within the Outdoor Education Centre overall title, and despite the other changes involved, it remains in spirit the Sandwell 'Outward Bound' (type) School, however unofficial that name must be.

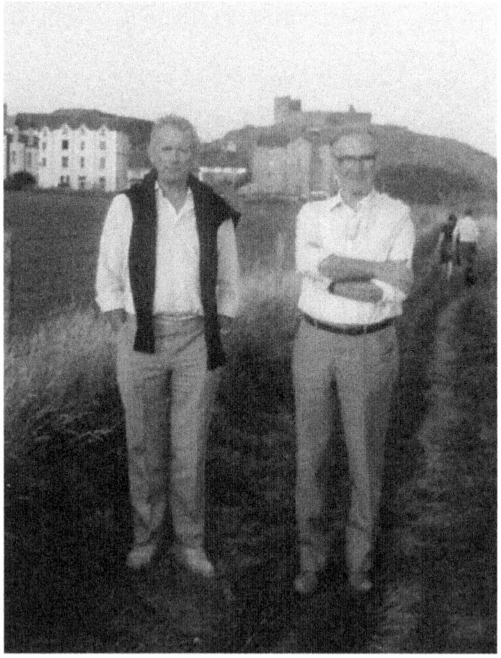

Murray Watterson with former Plas Gwynant handyman, Gene Diamond Both in retirement 1993

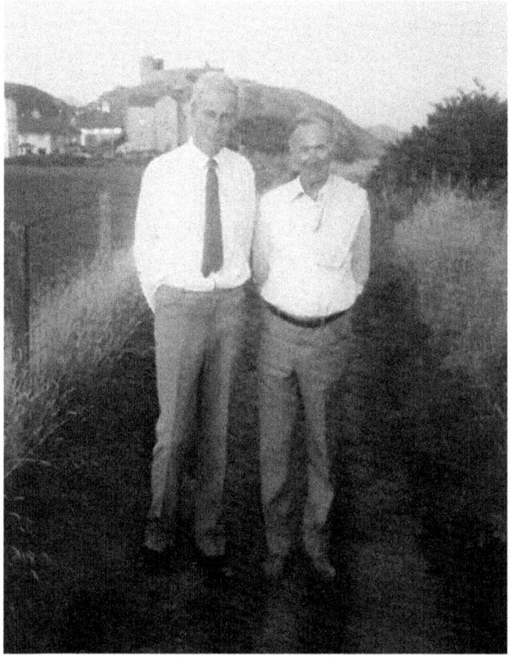

John Murden with Gene Diamond, Both photographs with Criccieth Castle in the background.

Patrick Belshaw – Sandwell Local Education Authority

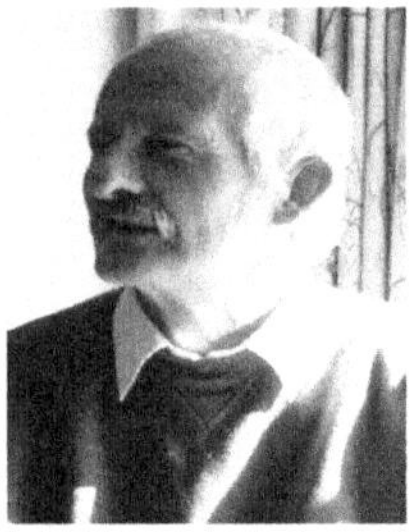

Patrick Belshaw's connection with Plas Gwynant was through Sandwell LEA, where from 1976 - 1980 he was a General Adviser, with a number of specialisms, including Outdoor Education. In this capacity, he carried an educational brief, where John Murden had the administrative brief for all of Sandwell's Centres, including Plas Gwynant and the Standing Camp at Bracelands. Patrick writes:

The Head of Plas Gwynant at that time was Murray Watterson, who was awarded the OBE for his services to outdoor education, much I think to his surprise (even slight embarrassment!) I continued to have some contact with him after I joined HM Inspectorate in 1980, and I was delighted to see that the work at Plas, which originally had an 'outward bound' feel to it (and for boys only!) was moving on to embrace a broader concept of outdoor education.

~ THE FIRST COURSES AT PLAS GWYNANT ~

It is important to include the experiences of those who attended Plas Gwynant and none more so than the very first pioneering intake in 1958.

Included here are some extracts from the pamphlet produced by Mr John Murden for Sandwell Department of Education 'Plas Gwynant The First 25 Years 1958-1983'.

John Murden, Deputy Director of Education (1983)

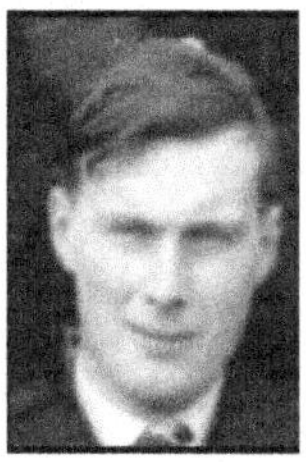

Friday 16 May 1958. Looking back, it seems a long time ago. Little did we all realise that we were making history as we boarded the coach at Hill Top Secondary Modern School for Boys. Thirty boys under the leadership of Mr Jack Lowe (later Deputy Head, Wodensborough High School) were going as the first party of West Bromwich pupils to camp at a new camp site at Plas Gwynant. On arrival on the site we discovered that only by boiling water from the stream was it possible to get drinking water. The instruction booklet had said 'Do not expose yourself to the sun all day', as it happened there was little chance as it rained every day of our time there. I clearly remember that we all learnt so much about our pupils. We thought we knew them, but a weeks' camping helped us all to discover things that we had not managed to find out in the classroom. We all learned to live together and realise there are always others to consider. The experience at Plas Gwynant is something which I have kept and have used to support Outdoor Education as a valuable part of the curriculum. It is not an extra which can be cut when finances are scarce and something must be sacrificed in terms of efficiency.

The highlight of the week was an ascent of Snowdon by Mr Lowe and Mr Gibbons – I realise now how amateurish we all were. They met a party from Hayes Comprehensive School, Middlesex. Two pupils were taken ill – a reminder that things can go wrong, and that planning is often overtaken by events and that common sense is necessary in all activities out of doors. The film 'Inn of the Sixth Happiness' was being shot in the area. On our expedition, we came across the Chinese film sets amid the Welsh mountains. Whenever I see the film I think of the wet days in Gwynant Valley, disguised cleverly on the screen – now the small TV screen.

The experience of living together and cooking our own meals was very valuable – the menus seem very dull and fattening today; although liver and bacon was very acceptable after climbing Snowdon. The week helped to put our lives into perspective and realise that passing exams is important but is not everything in life. The experience of sharing a tent, sharing chores and helping one another out of doors is an important part of growing up. Outdoor Education is now recognised as an important part of the curriculum.
This weeks' experience in 1958 helped *me* to realise the importance of this activity. Hill Top always were pioneers and I am proud to have been a teacher, the week taught me many lessons which I have *never* forgotten.

John Murden's Journal:

During the course, it was expected that everyone kept a journal, or diary, of their experience. Mr Murden was no exception! Below are the entries he made during his stay in 1958. Pupils were divided into groups – A, B and C, with their respective teachers, and again into groups of 5 and timetables set out.

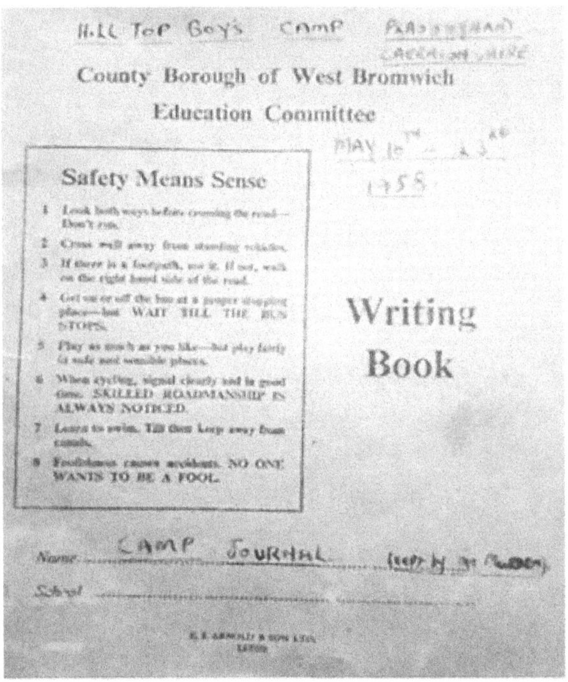

Hill Top Boys Camp Plas Gwynant Caernarvonshire

County Borough of West Bromwich

Education Committee

May 16th – 23rd 1958

Safety Means Sense

1 Look both ways before crossing the road—Don't run.
2 Cross well away from standing vehicles.
3 If there is a footpath, use it. If not, walk on the right hand side of the road.
4 Get on or off the bus at a proper stopping place—but WAIT TILL THE BUS STOPS.
5 Play as much as you like—but play fairly in safe and sensible places.
6 When cycling, signal clearly and in good time. SKILLED ROADMANSHIP IS ALWAYS NOTICED.
7 Learn to swim. Till then keep away from canals.
8 Foolishness causes accidents. NO ONE WANTS TO BE A FOOL.

Writing Book

Name: CAMP JOURNAL (kept by Mr Murden)

School

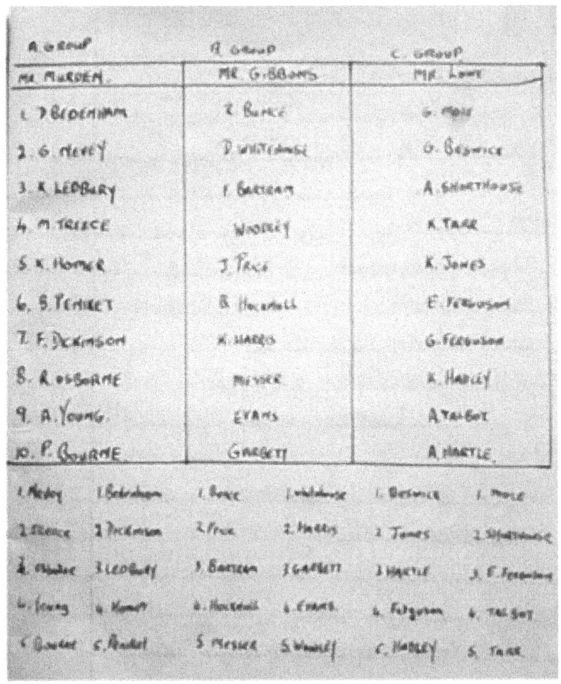

A. Group	B. Group	C. Group
Mr Murden	Mr Gibbons	Mr Lowe
1. T. Bedenham	R. Bunce	G. Mole
2. G. Mercey	D. Whitehouse	G. Beswick
3. K. Ledbury	F. Bartram	A. Shorthouse
4. M. Treece	Woodley	K. Tarr
5. K. Homer	J. Price	K. Jones
6. S. Pennett	B. Hocknell	E. Ferguson
7. F. Dickinson	K. Harris	G. Ferguson
8. R. Osborne	Messer	K. Hadley
9. A. Young	Evans	A. Talbot
10. P. Bourne	Gargett	A. Hartle

1. Mercey	1. Bedenham	1. Bunce	1. Whitehouse	1. Beswick	1. Mole
2. Treece	2. Dickinson	2. Price	2. Harris	2. Jones	2. Shorthouse
3. [illegible]	3. Ledbury	3. Bartram	3. Gargett	3. Hartle	3. E. Ferguson
4. Young	4. Homer	4. Hocknell	4. Evans	4. Ferguson	4. Talbot
5. Bourne	5. [illegible]	5. Messer	5. Woodley	5. Hadley	5. Tarr

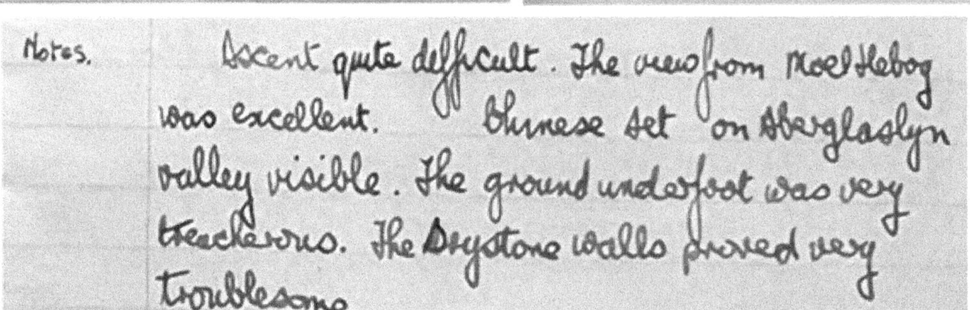

Notes. Ascent quite difficult. The view from Moel Hebog was excellent. Chinese set on Aberglaslyn valley visible. The ground underfoot was very treacherous. The drystone walls proved very troublesome.

General Time Table

Friday Arrived 1.30 Dinner 6.30.
Supper 9.15

Sat A. B- Moel Hebog (no gibbons)
C- Aberglaslyn Falls (no [illegible])

Sun B A- Gladstone rock (a.m.) Beddgelert Village
return by lake [illegible] (p.m.) – no gibbons
C- [illegible] – no Marsden

Mon C A+B- Beddgelert and Moel Hebog – no gibbons
and no Marsden.

Tue A C+B [illegible]
[illegible]

Wed [illegible]
down Pyg track

Thurs General tidy up.

CAMP TIME TABLE

7am	Duty Group Reveille
7.30	General Reveille
8am	Breakfast
8.30 - 9am	Tent + Camp Tidying
9.am	Tent inspection
9.10	Assembly
9.20-30	Bank
9.30	Set off
9.45	Duty Party Report for Work
1.pm	Lunch
4.15 pm	Afternoon Tea
6.30pm	Dinner
7.30	Shop Open
9pm	Supper
9.45	Prayers Lights Out.

WEATHER

Friday 6pm 57° 8pm 49°
Misty to the north. Clear sky at night. Venus seen. Windy variable.

Saturday 8am 47° 12noon 53° 4pm 66° 8pm 56°
Rain 28cc
It rained all morning. Misty to the the North. The weather improved in afternoon and the evening was cool and misty with only a light breeze.

Sunday 8am 47° 12noon 50° 4pm 56° 8pm 50°
Rain 37cc
It rained in the morning and heavily at night. The mist still persisted. Wind very strong at times, mostly from North. Humidity high.

Monday 8am 48° 12noon 55° 4pm 58° 8pm 50°
It rained periodically all day. Sometimes it was merely misty rain at other times it poured down.

Rain 20cc
The wind again was strong, especially at night. The direction was westerly.

Tuesday 9am 57° 12noon 56° 4pm 55° 8pm 49°
Early in the morning it was warm but a cool breeze reduced temperature. Rain came at 5.30 and continued at irregular intervals all night. The wind was strong at times. Snowdon was completely covered with mist. Beaufort Scale 1.
Rain 10cc
11.30pm 50°

Wednesday 6am 47° 9am 58° 12noon 60° 4pm 64°
8pm 58° 9.30pm 56° Max Temp 67° (2pm)
Rain 8cc
Rainfall early in the morning, but the day was the best so far. The sunny periods were cooled by cool breezes. Snowdon was clearly visible at times. The mist descended at night.

Monday Parties A+B went to Beddgelert by road; then ascended the west face of Moel Hebog, from Aberglaslyn Valley.
They returned through Parc Tyn-y-coed forest to Caernarvon road, below old camp site. They returned through Beddgelert village.

Menus recorded, as well as flowers and birds seen.

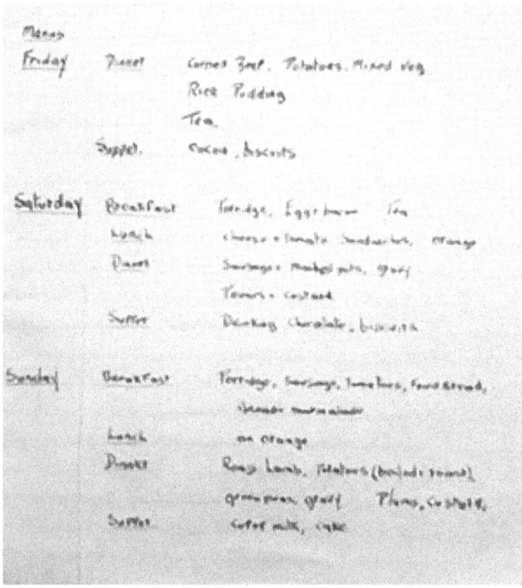

Menus

Friday Dinner Corned Beef, Potatoes, Mixed Veg.
Rice Pudding
Tea.
Supper. Cocoa, biscuits

Saturday Breakfast Porridge, Egg + bacon Tea
Lunch Cheese + tomato sandwiches, orange
Dinner Sausages + mashed pots, gravy
Prunes + custard
Supper Drinking chocolate, biscuits

Sunday Breakfast Porridge, Sausage, tomatoes, fried bread, [illegible] marmalade
Lunch an orange
Dinner Roast Lamb, Potatoes (boiled + roast), green peas, gravy Plums, custard.
Supper Coffee milk, cake

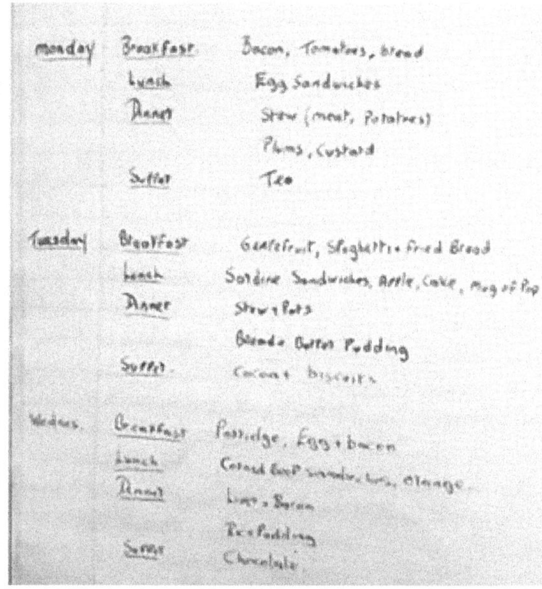

Monday Breakfast Bacon, Tomatoes, bread
Lunch Egg Sandwiches
Dinner Stew (meat, Potatoes)
Plums, Custard
Supper Tea

Tuesday Breakfast Grapefruit, Spaghetti + fried Bread
Lunch Sardine Sandwiches, Apple, Cake, Mug of Pop
Dinner Stew + Pots
Bread + Butter Pudding
Supper Cocoa + biscuits

Wednes. Breakfast Porridge, Egg + bacon
Lunch Corned Beef sandwiches, Orange
Dinner Liver + Bacon
Rice Pudding
Supper Chocolate

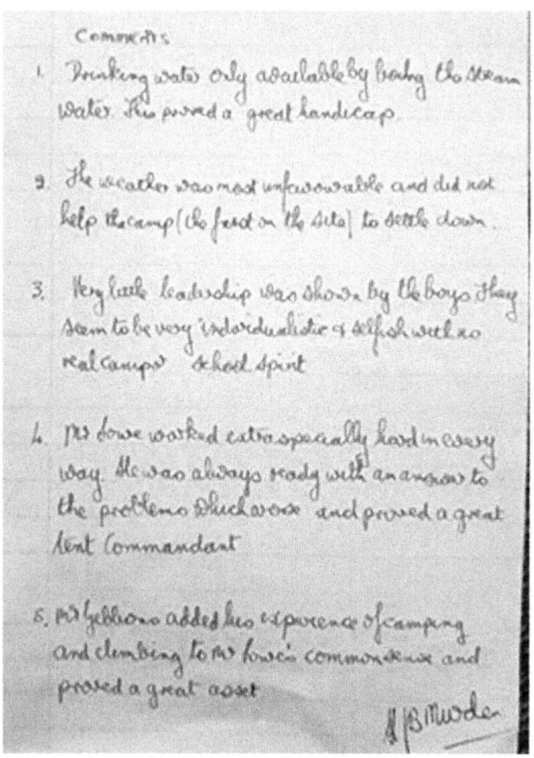

Comments

1. Drinking water only available by boiling the stream water. This proved a great handicap.

2. The weather was most unfavourable and did not help the camp (the first on the site) to settle down.

3. Very little leadership was shown by the boys. They seem to be very individualistic & selfish with no real camp or school spirit.

4. Mr Lowe worked extra specially hard in every way. He was always ready with an answer to the problems which arose and proved a great Tent Commandant.

5. Mr Gibbons added his experience of camping and climbing to Mr Lowe's commonsense and proved a great asset.

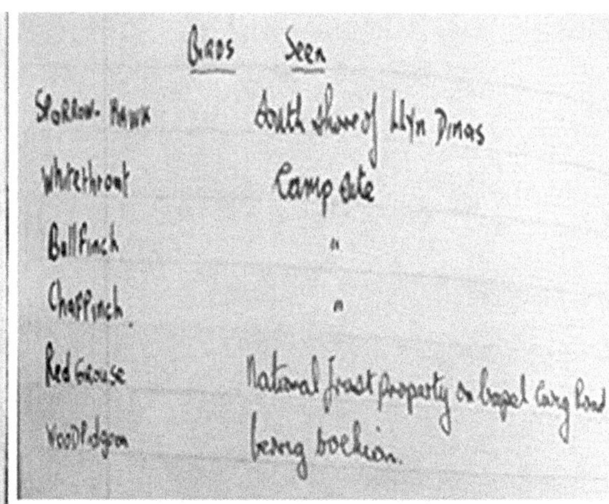

Birds Seen

Sparrow-Hawk South shore of Llyn Dinas
Whitethroat Camp site
Bullfinch "
Chaffinch "
Red Grouse National Trust property on Capel Curig Road
Wood Pigeon being [illegible].

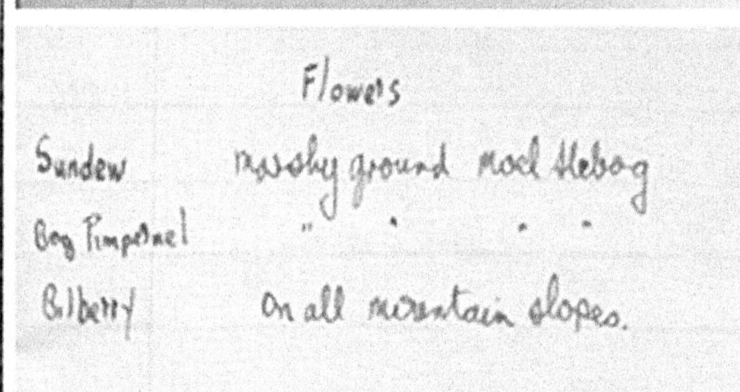

Flowers

Sundew marshy ground Moel Hebog
Bog Pimpernel " " "
Bilberry On all mountain slopes.

The 1958 Plas Gwynant Pilot Course

The first course to attend Plas Gwynant set off from Hill Top Secondary Modern School, with selected boys from several schools in the West Bromwich area.

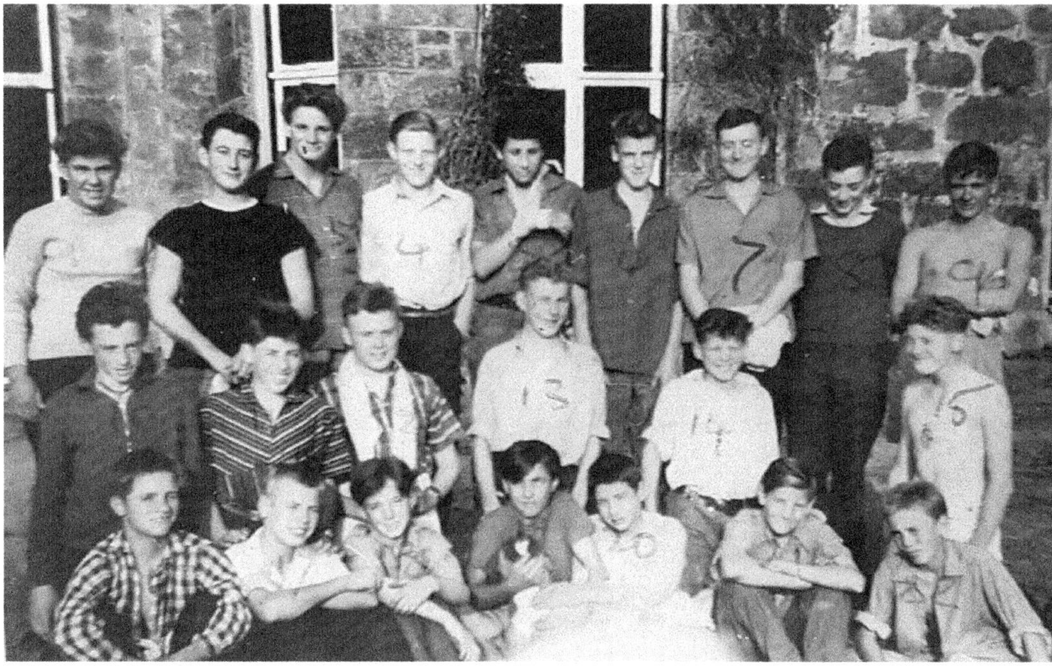

1958 Plas Gwynant Pilot Course No. 1 (in three Patrol groups)
Hunt: Tony Cail, Ray Cartwright, Nick Fisher, R Nixon, Mike Page, Harry Tandy, N Tarr, M Walton and D Wedgbury
Hilary: Cyril Corns, Walter Gough, J Whitehouse, C Middleton, J Molloy, J Morris and M Shenton.
Tenzing: C Bytheway, Eddie Hannington, M Jones, A Pincher, B Sherma, R Smith and A Wall

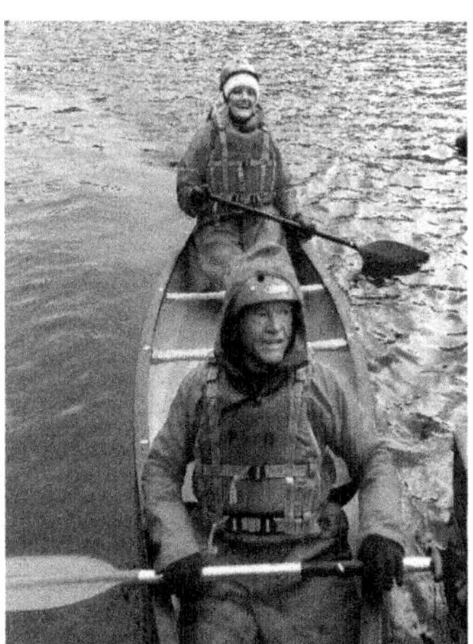

One member from this first photograph is Walter Gough (Wally), numbered 14 in the First Pilot Course picture above, who had been exceptional at Physical Training at George Salter Secondary Modern School for Boys and his reward was a place on the pilot course at Plas Gwynant.

Wally continues to attend the annual reunions for those who attended during the 1950s, 60s and 70s, and is pictured left with Judith Rogers.

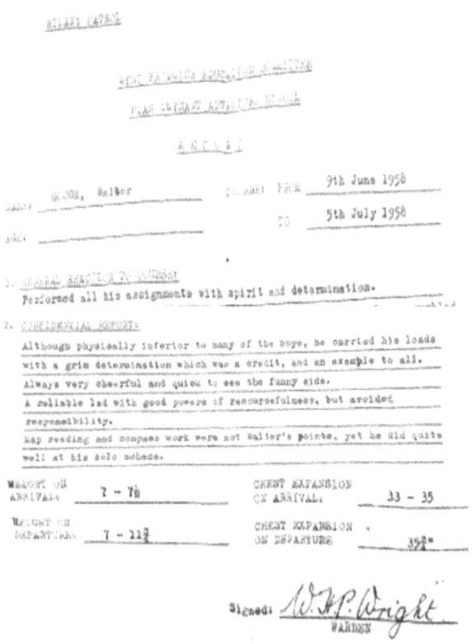

→

Hilary Patrol

West Bromwich Education Committee, Plas Gwynant Adventure School

REPORT

Name: GOUGH, Walter Course: From: 9 June 1958

Age: To: 5 July 1958

1.GENERAL REACTION TO COURSE:

Performed all his assignments with spirit and determination.

2.CONFIDENTIAL REPORT:

Although physically inferior to many of the boys, he carried his loads with a grim determination which was a credit and an example to all. Always very cheerful and quick to see the funny side. A reliable lad with good powers of resourcefulness, but avoided responsibility. Map-reading and compass work was not Walter's points, yet he did quite well at his sole scheme.

Weight on Arrival 7-7½ Chest Expansion on Arrival 33-35

Weight on Departure 7-11¾ Chest Expansion on Departure 35¾

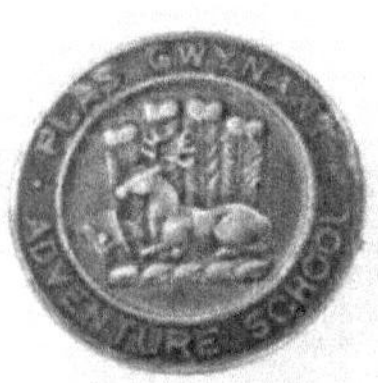

Wally Kept his report and badge after completing the course, where he had been given the responsibility for the upkeep of the Tilley lamps. He was keen to point out that the negative comments in the above report about map reading and 'avoiding responsibility' was totally untrue, as he excelled in both! He thinks that a certain pillow fight with his friends, which burst the feather pillows, left him out of favour with Mr Wright, the Warden! However, Wally's weight and chest expansion had increased, due to fresh air, exercise and good food.

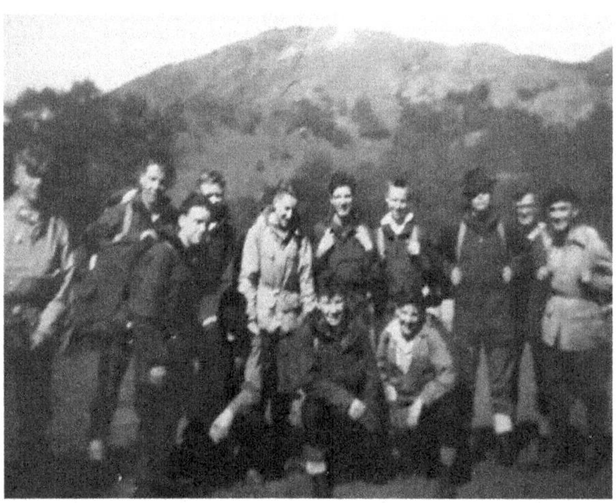

Wally's photograph from the first Pilot Course at Plas Gwynant: he is on the left at the front (side view, standing). Just behind him and second from left, is Cyril Corns. First left is Tony Cail. Others identified are: first right - name forgotten but this boy ended up in hospital after injuring his foot with an axe while chopping wood. Second right is instructor Mr Hughes. Third from right wearing a hat is Ray Cartwright who is 14 years old, but looks more like an adult. (Ray had forgotten to bring his hat and had written to ask his brother to bring it to him. His brother cycled all the way to Plas Gwynant from West Bromwich with his brother's hat, then turned right around and cycled back!) Fourth from right is Harry Tandy, who Wally thinks went to Churchfields School. And lastly, fifth from right at the back is a boy called Nick Fisher, who went on to become a footballer.

These diary entries (written by Gary Rushton) shows the write-up for his Map reading hike, the tin cans along their route gave clues about where the next can will be. Patrols record the time they discover each can, which have names such as borogove, gimble, wabe, etc., all taken from the nonsense poem 'Jabberwocky' by Lewis Carroll.

SATURDAY 21st APRIL

Awoke at 4:30 am but stayed in sleeping bags till 5:00. After cooking breakfast in darkeness we broke camp and set off at 7:30 am. We went to Pen-y-Pass along track and then climbed ridge behind hotel to outlet of Llyn cwm-y-ffynnon (BRILLIG-800 am). We got to Pen-y-Gwryd and then to the top of the knoll at 664552 (BOROGROVE-8.45). We got on to the main and walked to the milestone at 657526. Then we tried to follow the ancient trackway through Bwlch Ehediad to the ruined bridge at 678522 (GIMBLE-11.00 am). We retraced steps to main road and went to zig-zag path, half way along Llyn Gwynant. We ascended past the old house to the iron style (WABE-1.30). Then we made our way to spot hieght 790 but could not find a clue tin so sketched the summit. We returned through a "jungle" to Plas Gwynant being the first patrol to return. The house was deserted so we had showers when Ogwen returned they had 12 and Tryfan later returned having 11 because Dawes had hurt his ankle. In the evening we had inquisition to prove we had been to clue points. We estimated we had in the 2 days covered 35 miles and climbed 6,000 feet at least. Had letter from dad.

Clue tins recorded with times discovered. (From the diary of Gary Rushton)

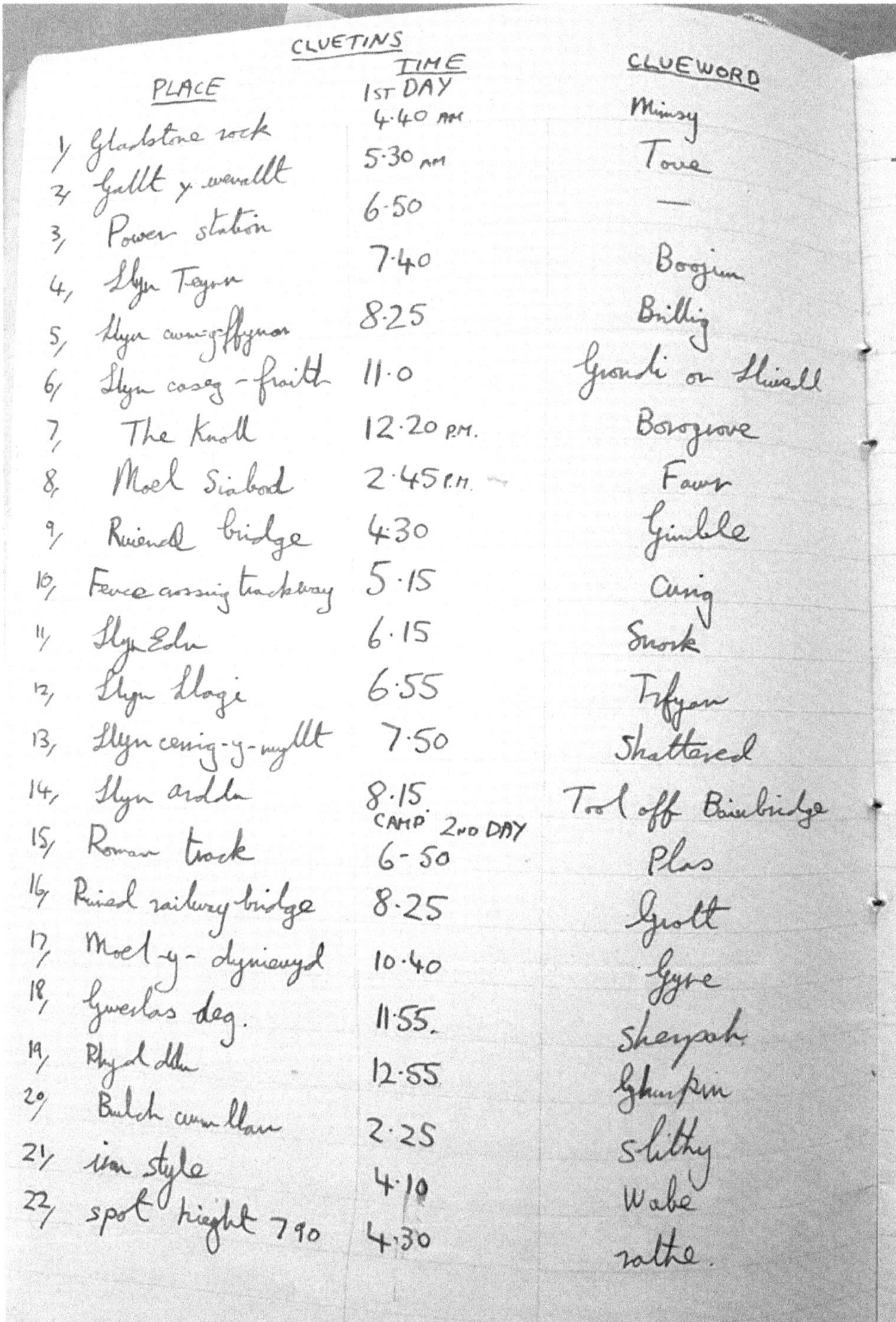

CLUETINS

PLACE	TIME 1ST DAY	CLUEWORD
1, Gladstone rock	4.40 AM	Mimsy
2, Gallt y wenallt	5.30 AM	Tove
3, Power station	6.50	—
4, Llyn Teyrn	7.40	Boogum
5, Llyn cwm-ffynnon	8.25	Brillig
6, Llyn caseg-fraith	11.0	Gronk or Llwall
7, The Knoll	12.20 P.M.	Borogrove
8, Moel Siabod	2.45 P.M.	Fawr
9, Ruined bridge	4.30	Gimble
10, Fence crossing trackway	5.15	Cwng
11, Llyn Edno	6.15	Snork
12, Llyn Llagi	6.55	Tryfan
13, Llyn cerrig-y-myllt	7.50	Shattered
14, Llyn adda	8.15 CAMP	Tool off Bainbridge
	2ND DAY	
15, Roman track	6-50	Plas
16, Ruined railway bridge	8.25	Gnott
17, Moel-y-dyniewyd	10.40	Gyre
18, Gwenlas deg.	11.55.	Sherpah
19, Rhyd ddu	12.55	Glumpin
20, Bwlch cwm llan	2.25	slithy
21, iron style	4.10	Wabe
22, spot hieght 790	4.30	rathe.

(More from the diary of Gary Rushton)

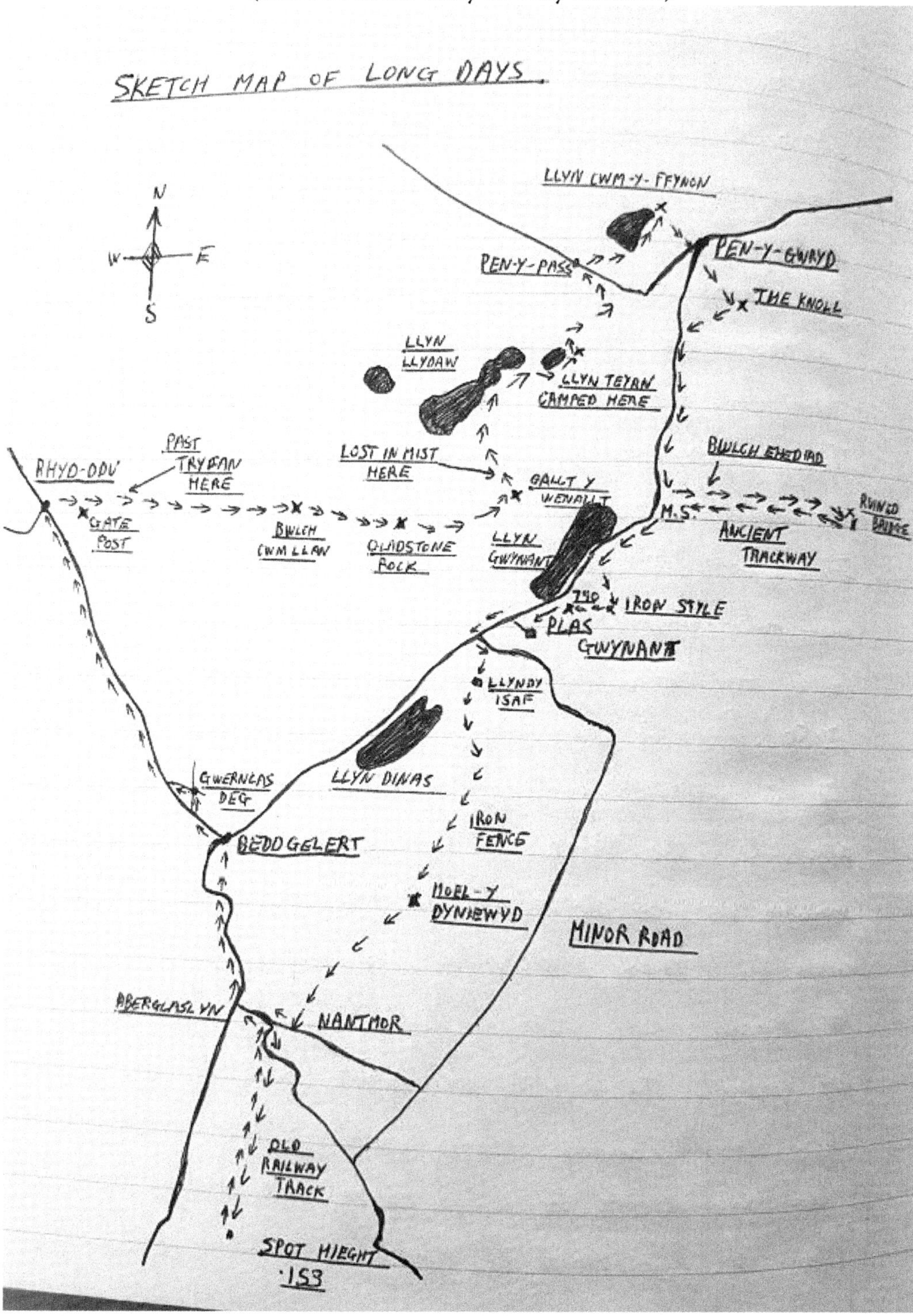

Eddie Hannington

Another boy who attended the first course was Eddie Hannington, who provided an account of his experience at Plas Gwynant in the pamphlet 'Plas Gwynant: The First 25 Years 1958-1983', which was produced by Sandwell Metropolitan Borough of Sandwell Department of Education. Eddie was Deputy Head Teacher at Cronehills Primary School 1970-74 and Head Teacher at Oakham Primary School 1983. He has also contributed a piece for this author's book 'The Cronehillians' which was published in 2013. Eddie writes:

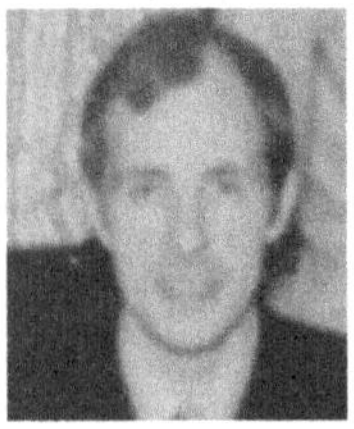

It was a very pleasant surprise to be chosen as one of the two boys from my secondary school to the new adventure school in North Wales on the pilot course. A month of 'outward bound' seemed most exciting, no one had been before, no one could tell us what to expect, no school-based folklore had been built up, we were not to be disappointed. The coach journey from Highfields to the Gwynant Valley seemed to take an age, but at last the gate was reached and at the end of the bumpy track was the house itself. It seemed small, isolated, and somewhat spartan in configuration. There was no electricity, no heating, save log fires, cooking was by solid fuel ranges, light in the evening was provided by Tilley lamps. What the building lacked in facilities was more than compensated for by the location and setting and the atmosphere which developed in that first month.

The staff for the pilot course consisted of the warden, Mr W H P (Bert) Wright, instructors Mr Pat Tweedale, Mr G Hughes and Mr I Shepherd. A cook was in residence and all other functions and duties were carried out by the boys. We were grouped into two patrols, Tenzing and Hillary. The log fires, supplied from the forest, gave the evening entertainment of yarns, stories and songs an added attraction.

Each day followed a similar pattern. The patrol rose at 6.30am to set out on a short run to the river for an early morning dip. The water was always icy cold. Back to the school for washing, beds to be made, rooms tidied ready for inspection then breakfast at 8.00am. Certain jobs such as washing up, table-laying and potato peeling had to be performed and then the work of the day could begin. Lunch time provided a welcome break when everyone met, the afternoon was set aside for work and that was followed by the evening meal. When all jobs were completed for the day, the evenings were for leisure, entertainments, diary completion and letter writing. Bedtime was 10.00pm and 'lights out' very easily effected by the staff.

One fateful Sunday morning resulted in Tenzing Patrol incurring a punishment for over-sleeping. The whole patrol had to run, clad in plimsolls, shorts and tops, halfway up the Watkin Path and back prior to normal duties and breakfast. Needless to say, having laboured body and soul in this fashion, and with the addition of the odd blister, no further incidents of late rising were recorded. Sunday was usually a day of rest, spent walking to Beddgelert, resting in the dormitory, reading or letter writing.

Leisure time gave us chance to explore the vast grounds, the stream, and the twin log bridge over the pool at the base of the waterfall. The barn always an attraction, its magnetic pull was two-fold. A colony of bats always made for interesting observation and the collection of medical books, deposited there following the death of the doctor who had previously owner the house. The books were old, musty, worn, but complete with illustrations of elephantiasis, 'berry-berry' and morbid facets of human existence such a fascination at this time.

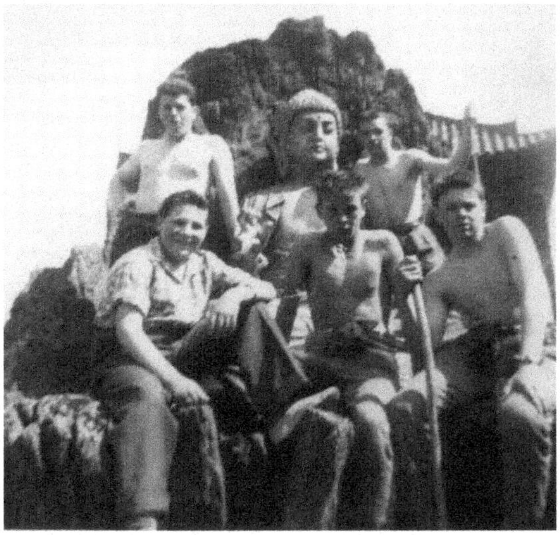

A favourite occupation was to walk to Llyn Dinas and watch the activities on the elaborate film set newly erected there. A replica Chinese village had been constructed for scenes in the film 'Inn of the Sixth Happiness'. Gladys Aylward, alias Ingrid Bergman, led the Chinese children to safety over the Welsh mountains!
Robert Donat occupied premises near to Plas Gwynant. Many of our rock climbs and mountain walks were punctuated by aircraft, making mock air attacks on the 'village' or involving themselves in dog fights for the purpose of the film.

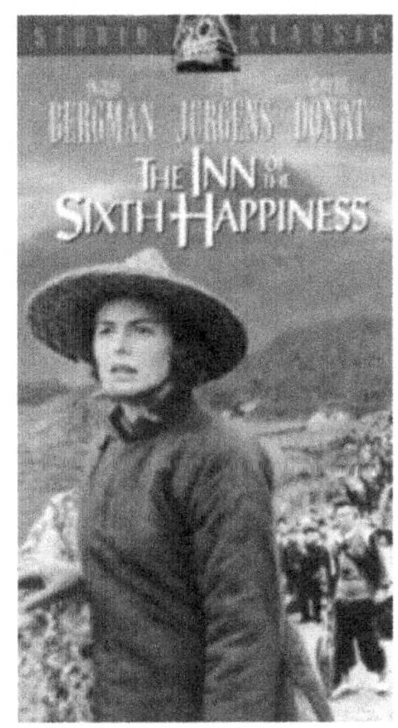

Every time a large saloon passed us on the road the same thought occurred – is it Ingrid Bergman? The famous film, directed by Mark Robson, won a Golden Globe Award for 'Best Film Promoting International Understanding' in 1958.

This true story was about Gladys Aylward (Ingrid Bergman), a British maid, believes that she is destined to go to China. She is rejected as a missionary, but she eventually finds her way to the town of Yang Cheng and happily runs an inn there. Her peaceful existence, however, is interrupted by Japan's invasion of China aided by Lin Nan (Curt Jurgens), a half-Chinese/half-Dutch military officer. Gladys must lead a group of orphans to safety by embarking on a dangerous mountain journey.

Most of the children in the film were Chinese children from Liverpool, home to one of the oldest Chinese communities in Europe.

For the six days each week we laboured, and some of the activities were as follows: grounds maintenance, which included weeding paths with chemicals, raking gravel paths, pruning, tidying and generally making the area presentable. A whole session was devoted to knots, unfortunately after all this time I can only remember the bowline. Mountain rescue lessons were fascinating, especially the simulated emergency. The Thomas stretcher came out and with 'Smithy' secured to it, the whole unit was lowered from Eagle Rock, barrow boy method. The 'patient' survived but was shocked and was never quite the same again.

Abseiling was one of the more spectacular activities, again from Eagle Rock. Everyone had a go; thank goodness for slings and karabiners, the classical method was horrible. Canoeing was carried out on Llyn Gwynant, a deep glacial lake, where the water is very cold. Every member of my patrol capsized, most doing so deliberately, few doing so twice, it was so cold. A very exclusive Tadpole Club was established that year for capsized canoeists of Plas Gwynant. Compass work and map reading was very important to the course and of paramount importance on later schemes especially the solo scheme.

Rock climbing was at first nerve racking and later most exhilarating. It seemed quite inconceivable that certain rock formations could be climbed but we always did it. The forestry work was most varied. Work in the nursery on weeding was backbreaking, using small sickles which regularly needed sharpening. Chemical spraying was simpler! Tree felling was most spectacular but during the dressing of branches one boy had a nasty accident, requiring several stitches in his foot. He later completed the course with the rest of us, having had a large patch attached to his damaged boot.

The schemes were the high point, where skills developed earlier could be tested. Light-weight camping in the mountains is pleasurable but physically demanding. Traversing scree with a pack on can be harrowing. Occasionally falls resulted in 'bent' and 'dented' plates and dishes. Try eating a hard-earned meal from a bent plate. No Fairy Liquid either for washing greasy dishes – just icy cold water and a handful of lake-edged gravel.

The final scheme was a solo one. Each of us set off alone with iron rations and a bivouac. Several objectives had to be achieved and it was necessary to be back at Plas Gwynant within strict time limits. The weather was dreadful. My first night was eventful, the bivouac was pitched against a stone wall, and one end was blocked off with an anorak and pack to keep out the driving rain. In the early hours of the morning the wind backed, forcing rain into the open end of the bivouac, soaking my sleeping bag. Sleep was impossible, so I gave up, commenced part two of the scheme at twilight, and arrived back early but very tired and wet.

The course ended after four eventful weeks with the award of a special badge. It gave 'town' boys an excitement not previously possible; it developed a responsible attitude to other people and to an environment which can be extremely hostile. Much of that course is still vivid in my memory, faces of the other boys' familiar but many of the names escape me.

What an opportunity Plas Gwynant afforded me. It must have done the same for hundreds of other boys and girls from Sandwell, may it go on successfully for the next twenty-five years.

Extract from 'The Cronehillians' School Magazine 1959 produced by West Bromwich Secondary Technical School

The First Pilot Course 1958

Pupils Nick Tarr, D Wall, J Morris, Form 5
(All pictured in the 1958 Pilot Course photograph)

On our arrival at Plas Gwynant. A large house in its own grounds, we were issued with our kit for the course. Our next job was to make our beds ready for the night. As soon as tea was over, Mr Wright, the chief instructor told us what we were expected to do while we were there. The day started at half past six with a dip in the river which ran through the grounds of the school. A competition for the best kept dormitory was started and the next job was to get the dormitory ready for inspection by Mr Wright. Breakfast came afterwards, followed by prayers.

As soon as prayers were over the lessons started and included map reading, map making, knotting, canoeing, rock climbing, forestry, light-weight camping and mountain rescue. It was planned so that if we spent the morning at school the afternoon was given over to outside activities, or vice-versa. Dinner was at 1 o'clock and tea at six. After six the time was our own to do as we pleased until 9 o'clock, when it was time for our evening drink and at half past nine it was time for bed.

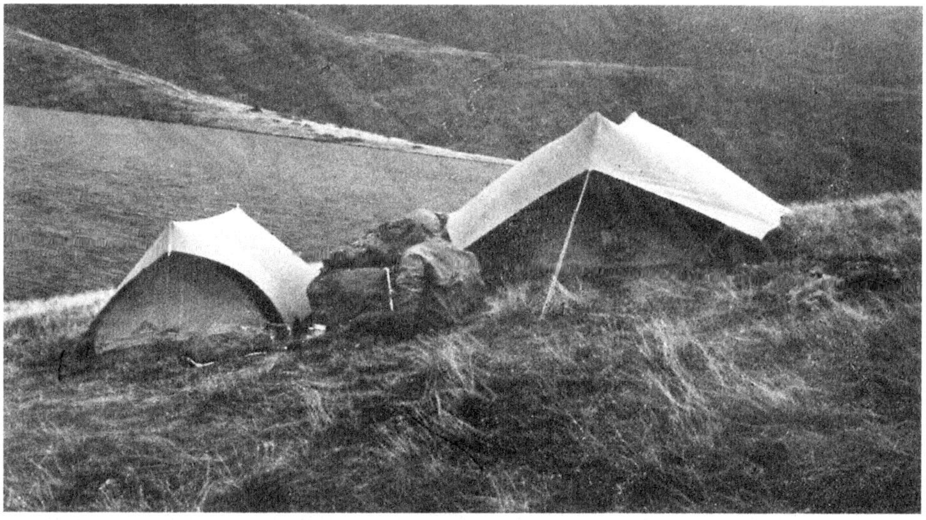

The part we enjoyed most was the schemes, especially the solo scheme, where we were sent on our own to spend the night in a bivouac sheet. As most of the boys put it, "It was murder!" All these things went together to make a most enjoyable month and to make it complete, Mr Wright decided we had all earned the badge of merit.

Michael Page Shares his Memories of Plas Gwynant Adventure School

(Another from the 1958 course and number 5 on the group photograph)

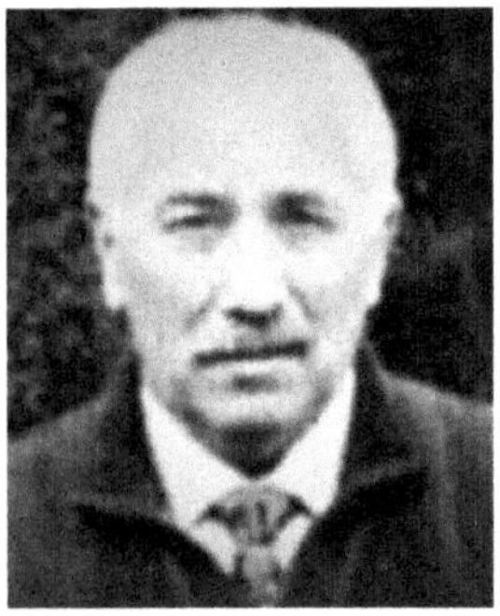

It was 1958 when I went to Plas Gwynant, though it was called Plas Gwynant Adventure School when I went. The first thing I remember was the bus forgot to pick me and one other from the school, so went up with the health inspector!

Early mornings was a bummer as you got out of bed, donned your swimming trunks with T- shirt and towel and jogged down the drive, turned left to the bridge over the river jumped into the freezing water for 20 minutes, then jogged back for breakfast - which was again funny as we were on the first course of the season and they had forgotten to send any plates and cups etc., so we used the camping utensils and one dish covered all. As you came out of the front door to your left down a small hill was an island in the stream where differences were sorted (which there was a few).

I am sure that when we went it was for around five weeks, but I know that shortly after they reduced the duration of the course. We did map reading and would go out with just a map reference and would stay out in the Snowdon area for two nights with either a tent or bivouac sheet which was just like a large sheet that you put on a wall held in place with stones and the ends open. I remember one morning I could feel something touching my feet thinking it was one the other boys messing about. I asked whoever it was to stop messing about, but when I looked it was a sheep grazing!

I was a patrol leader and one day we all went onto Lake Bala with the canoes. As a leader I had to make sure that everyone knew how to turn a canoe over and get themselves back upright. Everything was okay until the instructor realised that I was dry and had not been under (me being a non-swimmer) and thought I had got away with it - no chance, over I went.

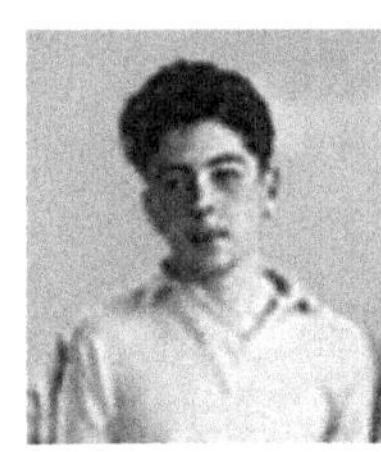

The climbing was great fun especially when you lost your footing and the natural thing to do is grab the rope (wrong) and you were left scrambling to get your footing. There was one time when we were climbing a thing they called the chimney which is two rocks with your back on one side then your feet against the other and would work yourself up. I was alright being tall, but the small guys had a big problem. But we all worked as a team and all got to the top. I had a sore on my side caused by a rucksack and the instructor said we could go to the hospital or they would treat it. So I said they could do it. They poured something onto it that bubbled up and hurt like hell, but cured the problem.

David Snell shares his memories of Plas Gwynant

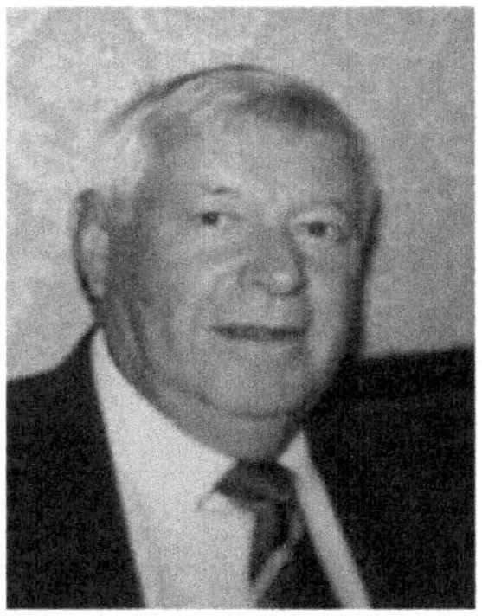

I went with a group from Beeches Road School; I think it was in the spring - possibly May, in the late 1950's. We were taken by coach and had a week there. I remember we were in ex-army bell tents in groups of six to eight boys. I don't remember any girls, but I also don't remember any of the boys either, sorry!

I was homesick, which started after one boy had been collected by his parents in a car. I realise now it was a state brought on by myself and didn't help me or the leaders who had to deal with it.

I do remember the stream on two sides and swimming or bathing in it. It was a whole new experience but ultimately very enjoyable although cold.

We walked up the Watkin path to the summit of Snowdon, stopping for sandwiches on some rocks on the way up. The weather deteriorated on the way up with rain and mist. I think there was some doubt about carrying on but the teachers decided to push on as it wasn't a downpour. But with a party of 11 year olds, probably wouldn't have been considered these days.

When we reached the summit it was lighter and drier, and we were able to go up to the very top, where the peak was in bright sunshine and we were above the clouds stretching like cotton wool all around with no cloud above us. It was a fantastic sight which I still remember to this day. But I remember nothing of the descent. There were photos taken that day, of which I remember 3 but can't find them! There was one of us sitting on the rocks eating, one of the group snaking high up the path towards the summit and another of loads of us at the summit.

I believe that another group went up Moel Siabod but I missed out because of my behaviour and which contributed to my brother not going from Beeches Road School.

The school kept a journal of the week which I think they still had at the centenary of the building of the school. You might be able to see these if the school allows.

The first Course for Girls - June Fletcher remembers the course in 1960

In 1960, I attended George Salter Secondary Modern School for Girls. I would read in the local paper, The Chronicle, about the fun the boys were having at Plas Gwynant Adventure School. I wondered why the Adventure School was just for boys. I approached my Head Mistress, Miss Lewis, to ask why the girls couldn't go to Plas Gwynant. She couldn't give me an answer.

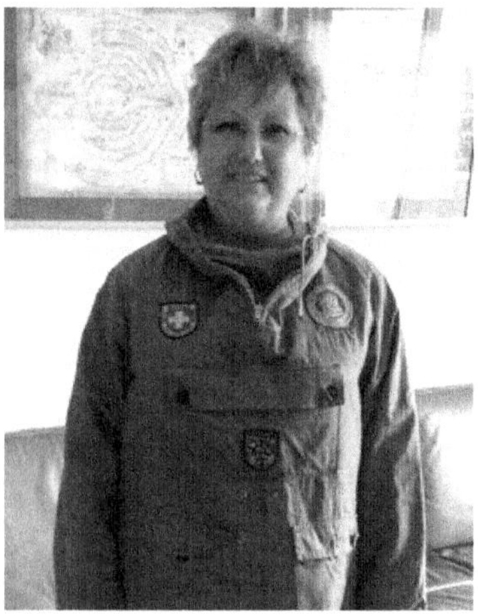

June models her 1960 Anorak
Below: June's anorak badge

A few days later she asked me and Carol Cooper to attend a meeting with her at the Highfields Building, in the Garden of Remembrance in West Bromwich. The meeting focused on whether the girls would be physically able to complete the four-week course. A week or so later Miss Lewis told us that there would be a girl's course but it would be a test course and slightly modified from the boys' course. Twenty girls were chosen from different schools in the area and we were given a list of supplies we had to buy, with instructions on how to prepare our feet so that we wouldn't get blisters.

The Anorak was made of heavy cotton and was quite water proof but heavy, not like the fabrics the gear is made of these days. Then came the boots. They were like big army boots, very heavy but surprisingly comfortable. I wore them for a few years.

We arrived at Plas Gwynant not really knowing what we were getting in to. The first thing was introductions to the group leaders. I remember Scotty Dwyer, Martin Endicote and Martin Riley. (Oh, Martin Riley; we all had a crush on him, he was so handsome). Then we were assigned groups - I was in the Tryfan group. Everyone settled in and we were assigned a 'job'. Mine was to keep the gravel pathways swept and tidy.

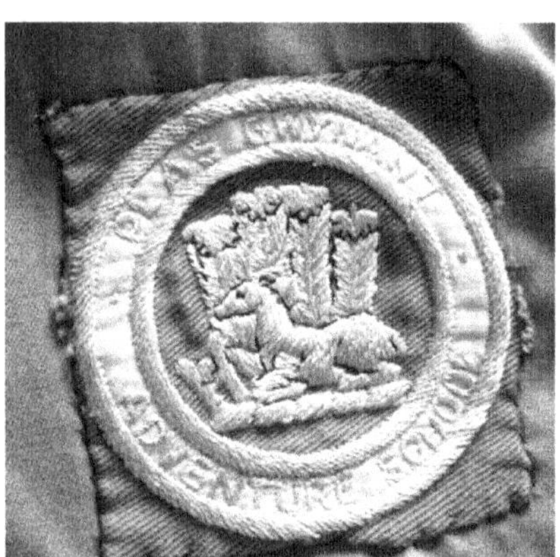

The days started early with in swim in the river - that woke you up! The girls were allowed to wear swim suits. You didn't hang around; the water was chilly. The only concessions that was made for the girls was that we were allowed to wear swimsuits; the boys swam naked! The last orienting exercise the boys would go out alone, the girls went in groups of four. Each day we learned new skills. Knot tying, map reading, learning how to use a compass. Then came the day when we went up to Eagle Rock to learn how to abseil.

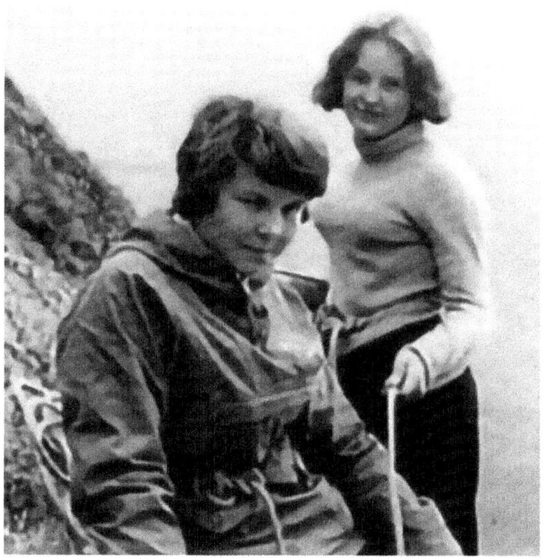

Above: Patty Condron on the left, June on the right

That rock appeared to be really high. Thirty years later, I went back for a visit to Plas; that rock wasn't anywhere near as high as it used to be! We learned mountain rescue techniques at Three Tree Hill, where you learn to trust your team members when you are on the stretcher - your life was in their hands. I really enjoyed the canvas kayaks that were lots of fun.

Then there was the orienteering. You were given a map and compass and a destination. The only instruction was not to hitch-hike. Well it was a long walk and a flatbed truck came by so we jumped on the back. Of course, we were seen and on arrival at the barn we were read the riot act! That night we slept in the hay, very itchy and the next morning we awoke to a very angry instructor.

Martin Endicote had driven his soft top sports car to the barn and the local cows found the soft top very tasty, they chewed the whole top.

We did a lot of camping in tents that were less than waterproof. The ground sheet was separate from the tent so everything could slip out. On one trip, the sheep got under the tent and ate our bacon on another it started to rain heavily and the water ran right through the tent everything was soaked. When I look at the light weight equipment you can get today I think back to the rucksacks we were given. They weighed a ton before you put anything in them. We carried everything on our backs, food, clothes cooking utensils etc.

Before we would set out there was a visit to the shed where the camp stoves and petrol bottles were stored. Each person was given a bottle of petrol and a stove. Gas went in one side pocket of our rucksacks and the stove went in the other. How did we ever survive?

I learned a lot during my stay at Plas Gwynant, I gained confidence in my own abilities to work as part of a team and to put trust in my team members. I truly believe that the experience and life lessons I learned during that one month in 1960 helped me throughout my life. The girls continued to attend Plas and I am proud that I was one of the 20 to take the first course and blaze the trail for others. I continued to climb mountains in Wales until my daughter was born. I have passed on my knowledge of outdoor pursuits to my three children who are now teaching their children. I still hike, canoe and kayak.

I live in British Columbia in Canada where you can pursue all kinds of outdoor activities, but I still hold Wales close to my heart. One day I will visit again.

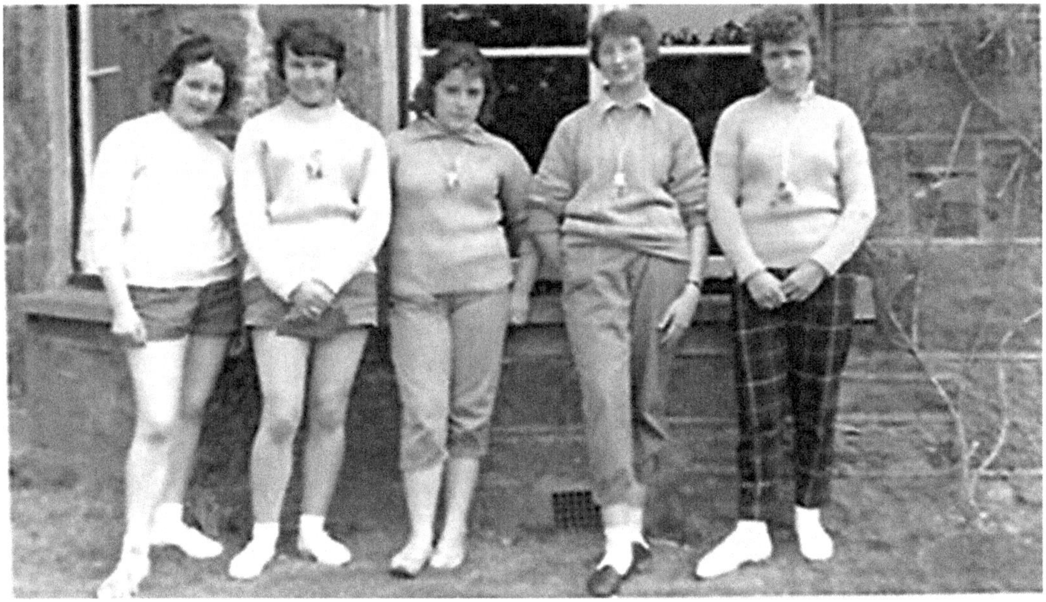

June Fletcher far left and Patty Condron is next to her.

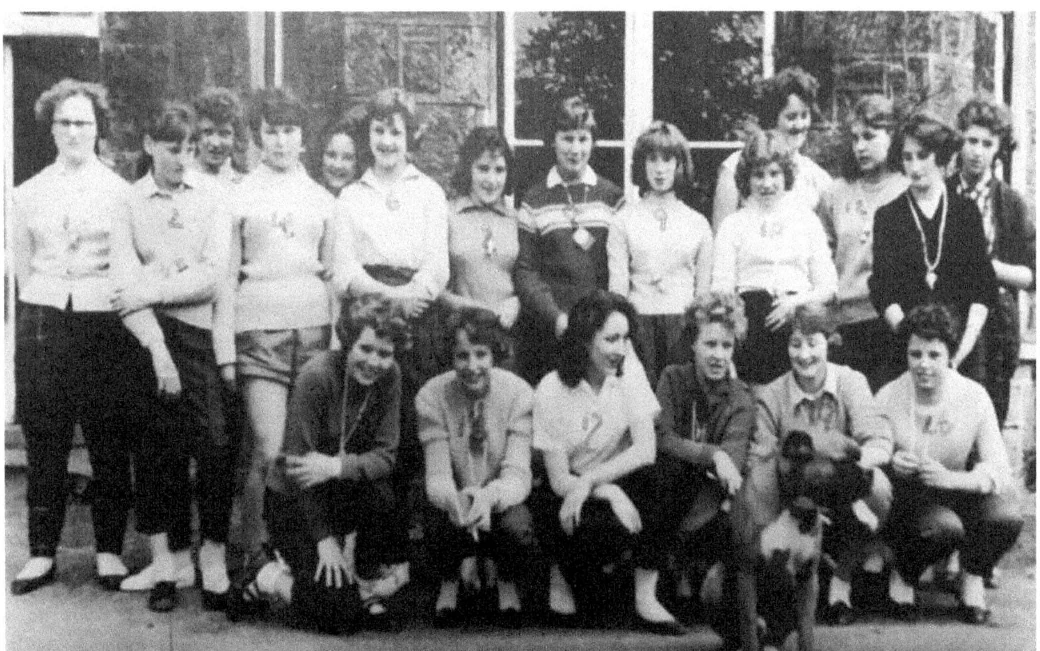

June is just visible on the back row - No.5 from left, Patty Condron is No.4

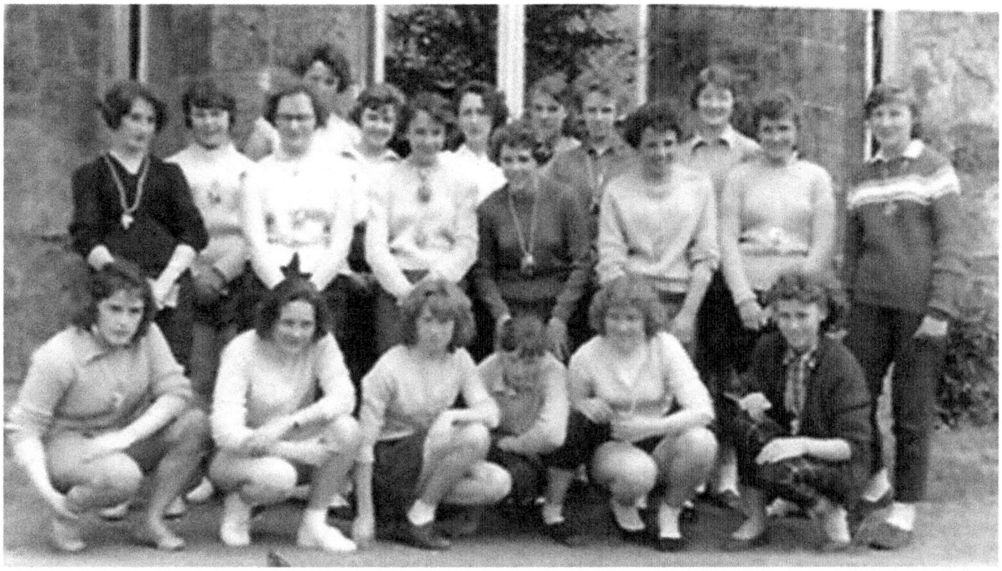

June Fletcher - Front row, 2nd left, with Patty Condron - 2nd row, 2nd left and Carol Cooper

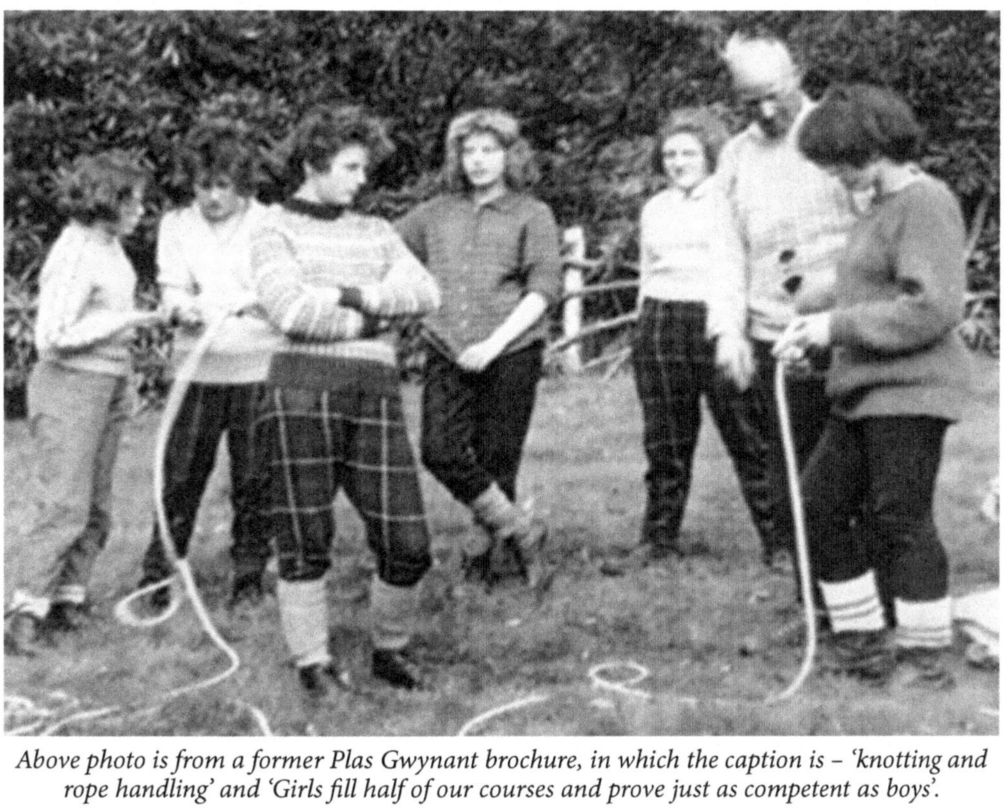

Above photo is from a former Plas Gwynant brochure, in which the caption is – 'knotting and rope handling' and 'Girls fill half of our courses and prove just as competent as boys'.

Pat Turton (nee Bye) shares her Plas Gwynant Journal

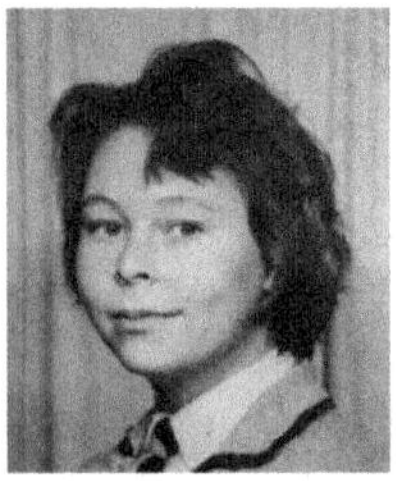

Pat attended All Saints Secondary Modern School.
Writing daily entries into a personal journal was part of the month-long course. Pat attended her Plas Gwynant course in April 1961, aged 14 and has kindly provided her red journal for inclusion here. Below are extracts from her hand-written pages; with transcript for easy reading.

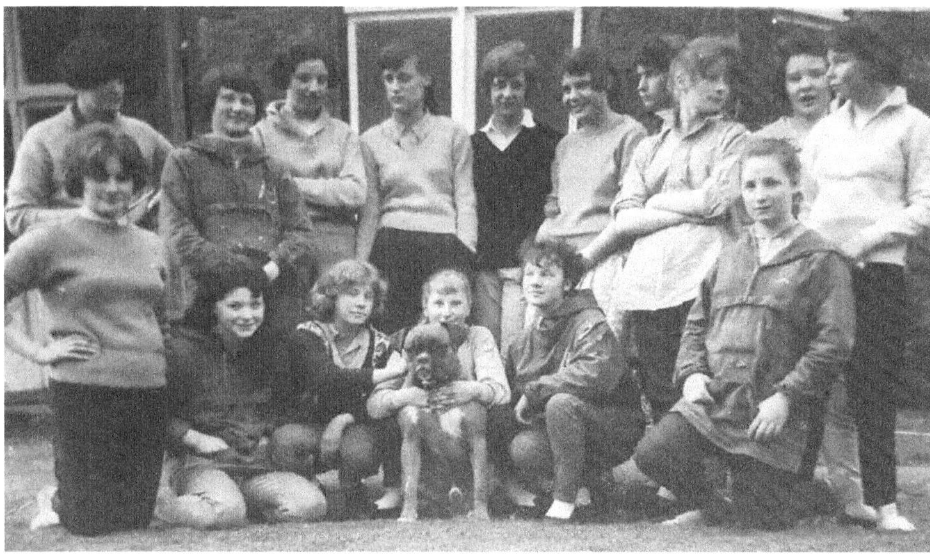

Pat is on the far right, standing

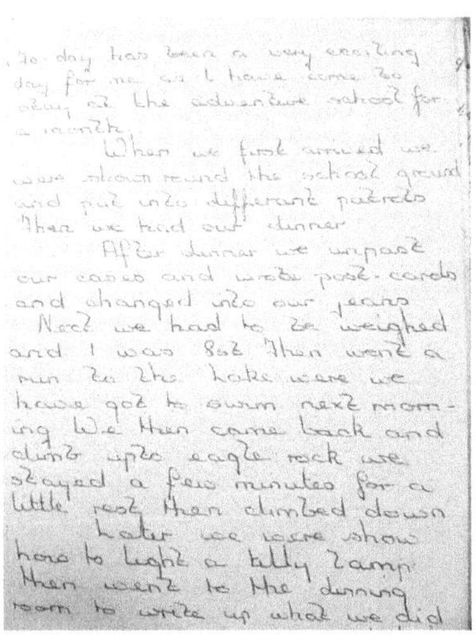

To day has been a very exciting
day for me as I have come to
stay at the adventure school for
a month.
When we first arrived we
were shown round the school ground
and put into differant patrols
Then we had our dinner
After dinner we unpast
our cases and wrote post-cards
and changed into our jeans
Next we had to be weighed
and I was 8st Then went a
run to the lake were we
have got to swim next morn-
ing We then came back and
climb upto eagle rock we
stayed a few minutes for a
little rest then climbed down
Later we were show
how to light a tilly lamp
then went to the dinning
room to write up what we did

Date: 3 April 1961
Today has been a very exciting day for me as I have come to Plas Gwynant Adventure School for a month. When we first arrived, we were shown round the school ground and put into different patrols. Then we had our dinner. After dinner, we unpacked our cases and wrote post cards and changed into our jeans.
Next, we had to be weighed and I was 8 stone. Then went on a run to the lake where we have got to swim next morning. We then came back and climbed up to Eagle Rock. We stayed a few minutes for a little rest, and then climbed down. Later we were shown how to light a Tilley Lamp. We then went to the dining room to write up what we did today.

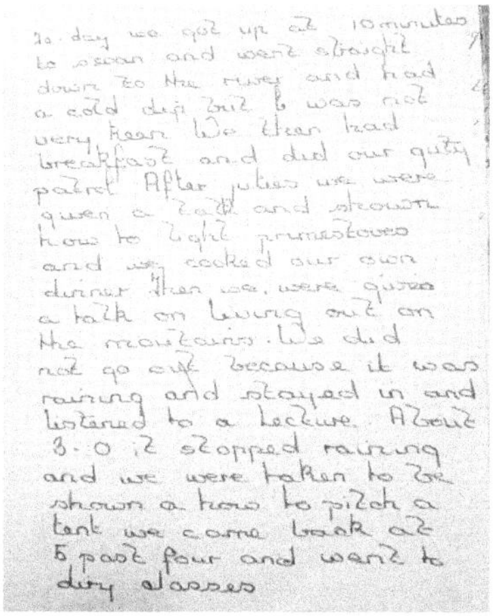

Date: 4 April 1961
Today we got up at 10 minutes to seven and went straight down to the river and had a cold dip but I was not very keen. We then had breakfast and did our duty patrol. After duties, we were given a talk showing how to light prima stoves and we cooked our own dinner. Then we were given a talk on living out on the mountains. We did not go out because it was raining and stayed in and listened to a lecture.
About 3 it stopped raining and we were taken to be shown how to pitch a tent. We came back at 5 past four and went to diary classes.

Date: 16 April 1961
We got up at 10 minutes to seven and went for our early morning swim. We came back, had our breakfast and did our duties. We then packed our rucksacks and set off to walk to Ogwen. We set off at 11.30 and reached Ogwen about 6.

We slept in a barn for the night and it was very comfortable. My friend Dorothy Chater had brought her wireless and we played it most of the night. The Instructors slept in the other part of the barn so they did not mind us playing the wireless.

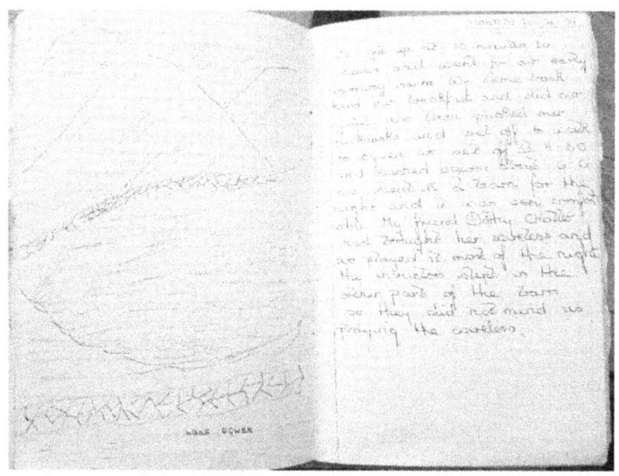

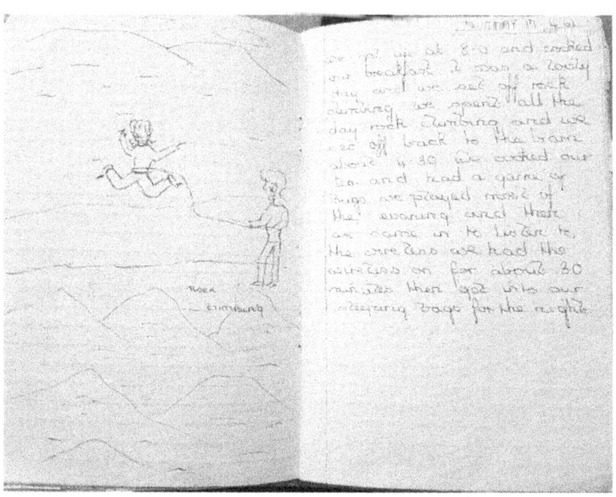

Date: 17 April 1961
We got up at 8 and cooked our breakfast. It was a lovely day and we set off rock climbing, we spent all day rock climbing and we set off back to the barn about 4.30.

We cooked our tea and had a game of Bugs. We played most of the evening and then we came in to listen to the wireless. We had the wireless on for about 30 minutes then got into our sleeping bags for the night.

Last Day – 27 April 1961
After breakfast, we did our duties and had inspection. After inspection, we had to give our kit in to Mr Dwyer. We then had morning break and did our test on the ropes. After the ropes, we had dinner then were given our option to write on the school. While we were writing, we had to go into the staff room for interviews. After interviews we had diary writing.

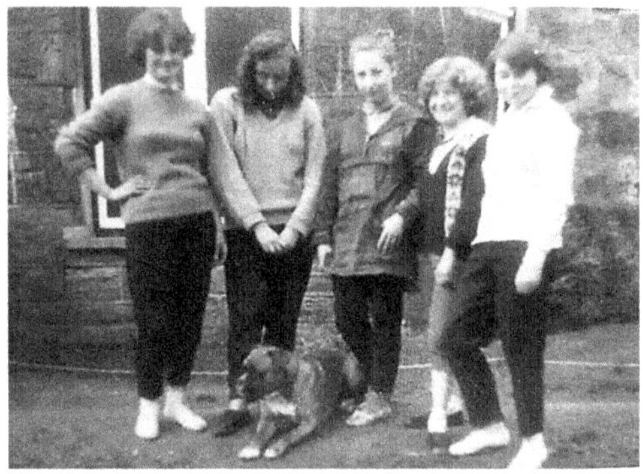

Pat Turton on the right

Pat Turton writes:
In the photograph below is me with 3 gentlemen taken in 2011 at the Plas Gwynant reunion; we had just finished canoeing (hence the wet suits). I also went abseiling over a 70ft rock aged 65yrs, doing the same exercise that I did age 14yrs. The gentleman who I am linking arms with is Philip Broadbent, who I had never met until 2011 when he and his wife came to view our bungalow that we were selling in Harlech. Philip at that time was looking to relocate from Lincolnshire. We started chatting about places we had lived and he told me he was born in West Bromwich and went to Cronehills High School, he was the same age as me. We continued to reminisce about West Bromwich and I told him about the Plas Gwynant Reunion that I would be going to in a few months, and yes, you may have already guessed, he had been on the course in 1962 also.

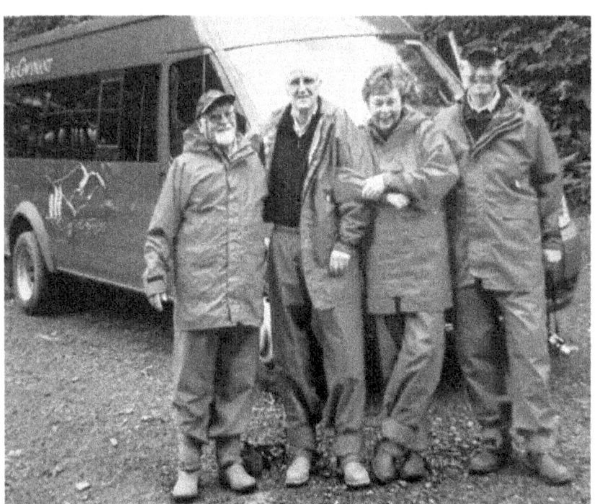

Centred are Philip Broadbent and Pat Turton at the Plas Gwynant Reunion 2011

He immediately booked a place, (after agreeing to buy the bungalow) and we both went off together, leaving his wife and my husband waving us off. It was a very enjoyable weekend, and although a lot slower, there was nothing I couldn't achieve that I had done when I was 14yrs old.

Brenda Murtha shares her group photograph

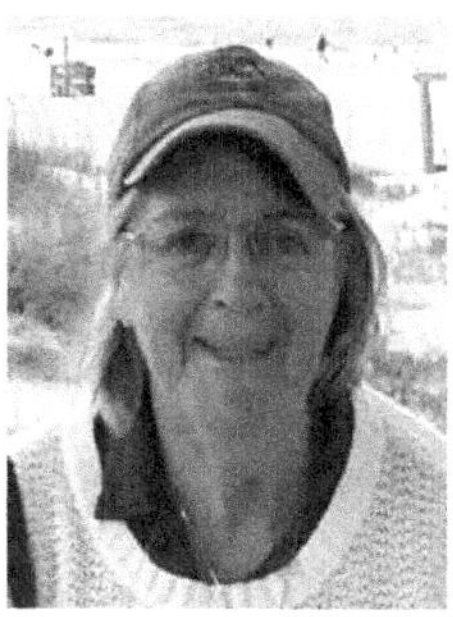

This is my group at Plas Gwynant, probably 1962 or 1963. I went to West Bromwich Technical High School and my name then was Brenda Osell.

My memories of Plas Gwynant - going on this adventure was a first for me, I was not an out of doors kind of girl. Since it was more than 50 years ago my memory may be a little rusty, the morning showers, the staff assigned to the shower room would yell and pull aside the curtain if they saw any steam coming from the shower. I was afraid of canoeing (still don't like it) I would paddle out just far enough to not get yelled at. Loved rock climbing, but had to get a shove of the edge to repel down. What I remember most was the last

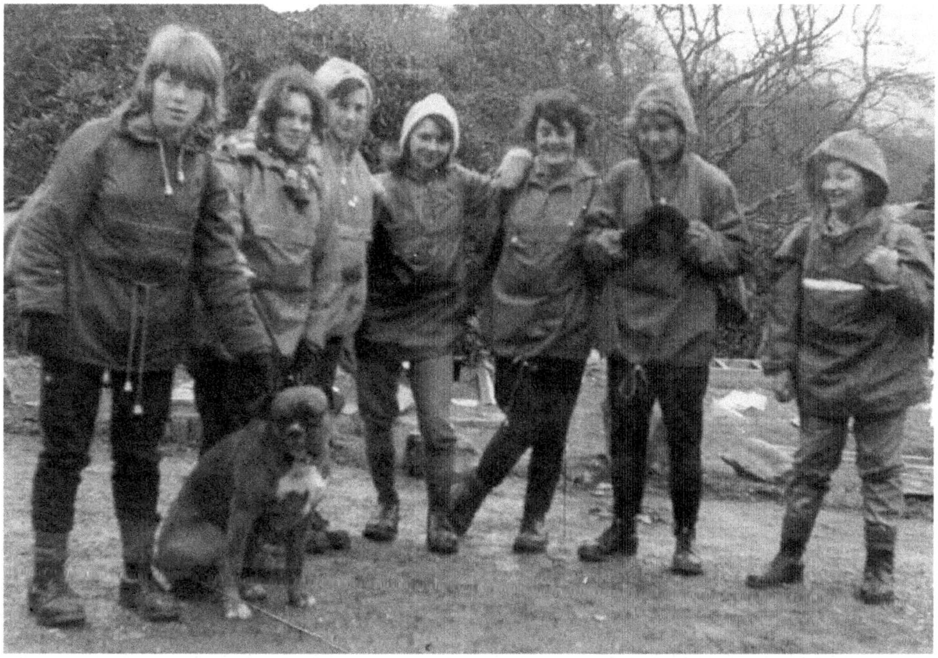

few days when we were sent out in groups for the overnight, we had to follow compass directions to get the clue on where to go next. If there was adult supervision I do not remember any. We were given a can of sweetened condensed milk, an apple and a chocolate bar (no campfires).

The upside of that experience I have been a Girl Scout for the past 40 years. Mostly as a troop leader for the past 30 years I have taught outdoor training to new leaders. I do not remember the names of all the girls in the photo, I think one was Veronica Vale (right) and another Christine, I am third from the right.

As I now live in the United States, sadly I don't think the reunion trip is possible in 2018.

Geoffrey Turner shares his group photograph

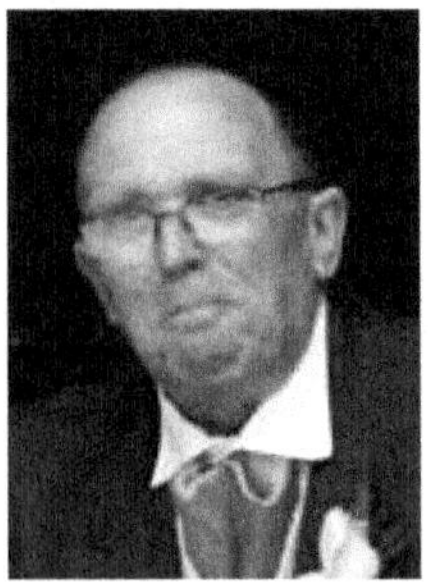

Boys just arrived from Charlemont Senior School, circa 1962 - Picture taken by their teacher, Mr Ben Graham.

Names include: Geoffrey Turner, who is sitting on the fence on the far left, Graham Pamplin, Ray Evans, Raymond Comerford, Billy Wallace, Tony Bradley and (?) Cookie.

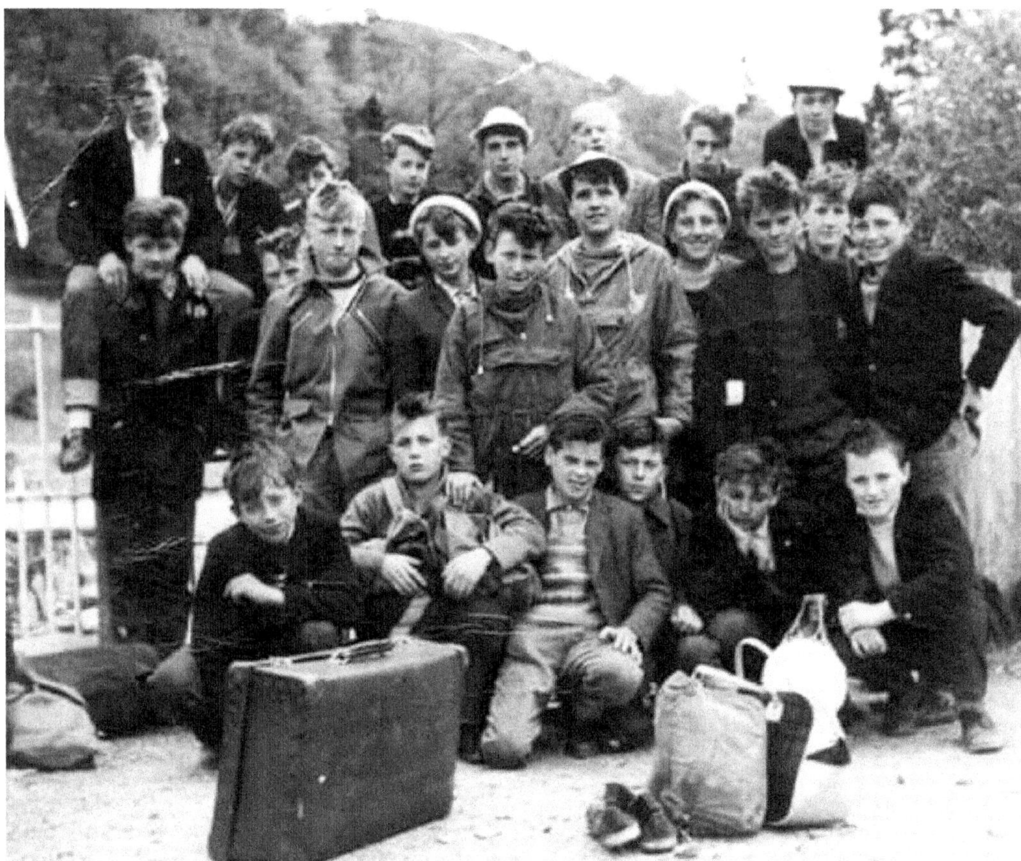

Advertising

Following the success of the Pilot Courses, the Education Department were keen to advertise

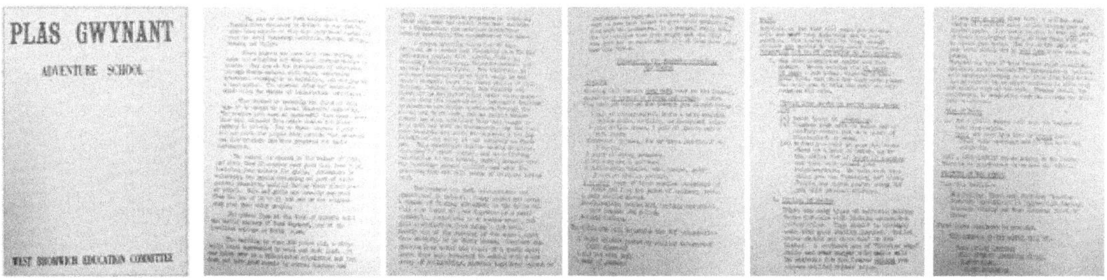
PLAS GWYNANT

ADVENTURE SCHOOL

WEST BROMWICH EDUCATION COMMITTEE

regular courses at Plas Gwynant. The following images are thought to be those of the first brochure with details of the course offered. (Brochure can be found at Smethwick Archives and is transcribed below).

Transcribed contents:

The idea of Short Term Residential Adventure Courses first developed in Britain in the 1940s. Since then schools of this type have been opened all over the world, including Australia, Malaya, Africa, Germany and Ceylon.
These courses are open to a wide variety of races and religions, but they have certain things in common. They aim at the development of the character through facing natural challenges, undergoing adventure, standing up to hardships and working as a team member, the course offers new interests which widen the choice of leisure time activities.

Plas Gwynant is possibly the first of this type to be opened by a Local Education Authority. The courses have been so successful that there have been many requests from other bodies for their members to attend. Two or three courses a year are set aside for people outside of West Bromwich and this brochure has been prepared for their information.

The school was opened in the summer of 1959 and since then 10 courses a year have been held including four courses for girls. Attendance is voluntary, the pupils attending as part of their general education, usually during their final year at school. Boys and girls are usually accepted from the age of 14 or 15 and one or two courses each year take older pupils. The school lies at the foot of Snowdon amid the varied scenery of Nant Gwynant, one of the loveliest valleys in North Wales. The building is some 200 years old, a stone built house surrounded by wood and park land. It was taken over in a dilapidated condition but has been put into good repair by course members and Staff.

A modernisation programme is under way which will make the school even more suitable as a headquarters for mountain activities without destroying the character of the place. A course normally lasts for 26 days, starting on a Monday and finishing on a Friday. Activities include hill walking, camping, canoeing, rock climbing, mountain rescue and various initiative tests. The timetable is arranged progressively so that early in the course students learn the basic skills of hill walking, camping, cooking, map reading and first aid on the lower hills under close supervision from the instructors. Intensive training in mountain activities continues through the second and third week and as pupils become fitter and more confident, they are taught to rely more and more on themselves. By the final week students are ready to organise a two-day expedition and carry it out entirely on their own.

This expedition covers nearly 40 miles, including 12 check points, and is a fitting culmination to the course, making demands upon the knowledge gained earlier, and upon the determination and willpower of everyone taking part. The courses are both recreational and educational in intent. Young people are given a chance of finding adventure in the hills and they also learn to live together in a small community, contribute to a common cause and gain satisfaction from doing a job well. Nearly all of the running of the school, apart from cooking, is in their hands. Teachers and parents have noted the value of a month spent here; boys have returned to school with a new sense of reliability, nervous boys have gained in confidence and boys who have never before done any work at home have helped to give their mothers a hand with the housework.

As a general rule, the fat children have lost weight and the thin ones have put on muscle while all of them have gone home much fitter.

Information for students attending the course

Clothing
Clothing will receive very hard wear on the course; therefore it should be strong and rough.
Apart from what you wear on the journey, you should bring:
1 pair of strong walking boots – with moulded rubber soles, or nails, as described below.
1 pair of gym shoes, I pair of shorts and 2 PT vests.
Underwear, Pyjamas, two or three shirts, 2 or 3 towels.
2 pairs of strong trousers.
2 sweaters and a pullover.
1 battle-dress blouse, wind jacket, golf jacket or similar article.
4 or more pairs of thick woollen stockings or socks and 1 or 2 pairs of ordinary socks.
1 pair woollen gloves.
Handkerchiefs, toilet kit, writing materials, boot brushes and polish.
Bathing costume.
The following will be useful but NOT essential:
1 light oilskin jacket or similar waterproof with sleeves.
1 old hat with brim and 1 pair of gaiters.

BOOTS
Blisters on the feet will cause you to miss work and apart from this they can be very painful. The course will be tough enough without you having to worry about blisters.

THEREFORE, PAY GREAT ATTENTION TO THE FOLLOWING:

1. Buy some methylated spirit and foot powder. Every evening for at least 14 days – rub meths vigorously into your feet and then dry dust with powder. The more you do this the more you will toughen the skin.

2. 'Break your boots in before they break you'
   a) Break boots in gradually.
   b) Toughen your skin as above and if chafing occurs, put on a piece of Elastoplast at once.
   c) Before you walk in your new boots stand in a bowl of water, up to the ankles for at least 10 minutes and then walk around your neighbourhood. Do this each time you are 'breaking in' boots. People may think you're crazy but you will prevent blisters.

Choice of Boots

There are many types of suitable walking boots for sale with Itshide or moulded rubber soles. They should be strongly made with good quality leather. Nailed boots should not have heel or toe plates.

A combined use of 'clinker Edge' nails and star rugger sole nails will be suitable for the course unless you choose moulded rubber soles. If you are in doubt about boots or nailing, seek advice at reputable shops selling camping gear and sports goods. You should be able to wear two pairs of socks inside your boots, so that these with you to choose your boots. The top of the ankle on your boots should not be more than 7 inches above the ground.

Whatever the type of boot (rubber sealed or nailed), the shoes should include two thicknesses of leather, each thickness running in one piece from heel to toe. What appears to be an upper thickness is often only the outside edge of the welt. Tongues should, for preference, be completely sewn in, to make the boots more waterproof.

Care of Boots

1. Rub a little dubbin well into the leather to keep it supple.
2. Never dry them by the fire or strong heat. Stuff with newspaper and let the boots dry naturally.
3. HAVE A GOOD HAIRCUT before coming on the course, there is no hairdresser at or near the school.

TRAINING AT THE SCHOOL

This will include:

Map reading, First Aid, Knotting, canoeing, Forestry, Expeditions in light-weight camping, Mountain walking and Rock Climbing, Mountain rescue. First class equipment is provided. Yours address at the school will be:

Name (BLOCK LETTERS)
Plas Gwynant Adventure School
Nant Gwynant,
Caernarvonshire
North Wales

COST

The cost of running the course is £40 per student. Transport is available free, to and from West Bromwich.

Derrick Lees shares his memories of Plas Gwynant 1962

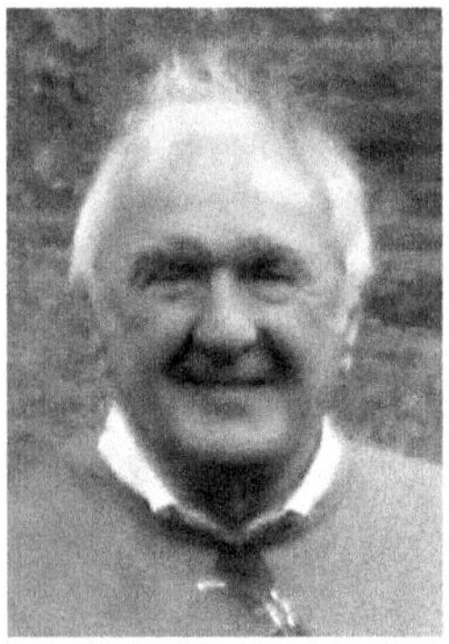

The first thing I remember was not long after arriving, one lad from Churchfields, whose name I think was Paul Schofield, after our normal evening chores, I heard him behind the school a bit upset. I asked him if someone was bullying him and he pointed him out; a lad I think from All Saints School.

The first opportunity to get him on his own was at the top of Eagle Rock, doing a mountain rescue exercise. I volunteered him to go in the stretcher all strapped in and volunteered myself to take the stretcher down. While passing through the bushes I asked him to stop bullying, to which he turned out a few obscenities – to which he received a Tipton handshake! He never bothered anybody after that. Paul was not a very good swimmer and he was paired up with me on a canoeing trip to Black Rock Sands. As we all know it was quite shallow water for a good way out, so out of devilment, I capsized the canoe and blind panic ensued until I told him to just stand up! (Sorry Paul).

I always wanted to go for a whole month to Plas after attending summer weekly camps in the bottom field where West Bromwich schools attended. The school stores, the old centre block where all the equipment is now stored used to be the chemical mixed toilet block to the left and behind it was where the toilets were emptied. As you can guess, it was my mate who fell head first into it – not a pleasant sight! There was also a rope course without safety measures or risk assessment back then.
I remember what was called the 'longest day' – a two-day course without any instructors. In other words, the team were on their own on their map reading course.

At the end of the first day we reached our destination by the bridge on the Nantmore back road. My team asked where we were going in the morning and I said, "up the shaving brush' whereby they said could they go up that evening to bivouac, and I agreed. I put my written note in a can under the pile of stones, as instructed by our tutor earlier in the course. We then made camp, but in the night the police and mountain rescue were called because we were not at our designated camp. I was summoned to the office and told off. I asked whether anyone had read my note – apparently not! But I still got my blue badge for completing the month.

Another thing I remember was my fear of heights, especially rock climbing in Ogwen Valley and abseiling down Eagle Rock, and I suspected the instructor knew this and was always pushing me to overcome my fear. Then there was the early morning run and wake up dip down by the bridge at the start of the Watkin Path for the strip off and totally submerge. A coach once drove over the bridge at the same time and hands were strategically placed to cover our embarrassment! I still hate cold water to this date because of this experience.

One evening we all went up the Watkin Path past the waterfalls to where the old slate cottages are on a very sunlit evening. Our instructor told us that, after pitching our tents, we were all to collect as many rocks as we could in half an hour and to split into two groups either side of the stream, a foot away from the edge. The object was to soak someone on the opposite bank - great fun before bedding down for the night.

A similar experience happened while in the Ogwen Valley in a barn which our beds were straw, but the evening was so hot that nobody could sleep and we were all playing up. It was then that the instructor, who could not get his sleep, said that we were to get up and strip off and go down to the stream at 2.00am in the morning and go right under in the cold water until everyone had done it, only then could they go back to the barn. Needless to say, the last six were thrown in so that we could get warm again and we all slept like a log that night.

Parents were allowed to come to Plas Gwynant half way through the course to see their children and spend the day with them and bring goodies from home. There was also a general store and post office over the bridge, which is now a private house, where we could all stock up on sweet supplies, etc., and then there was Beddgelert – what a lovely village; it is still one of my favourite spots.

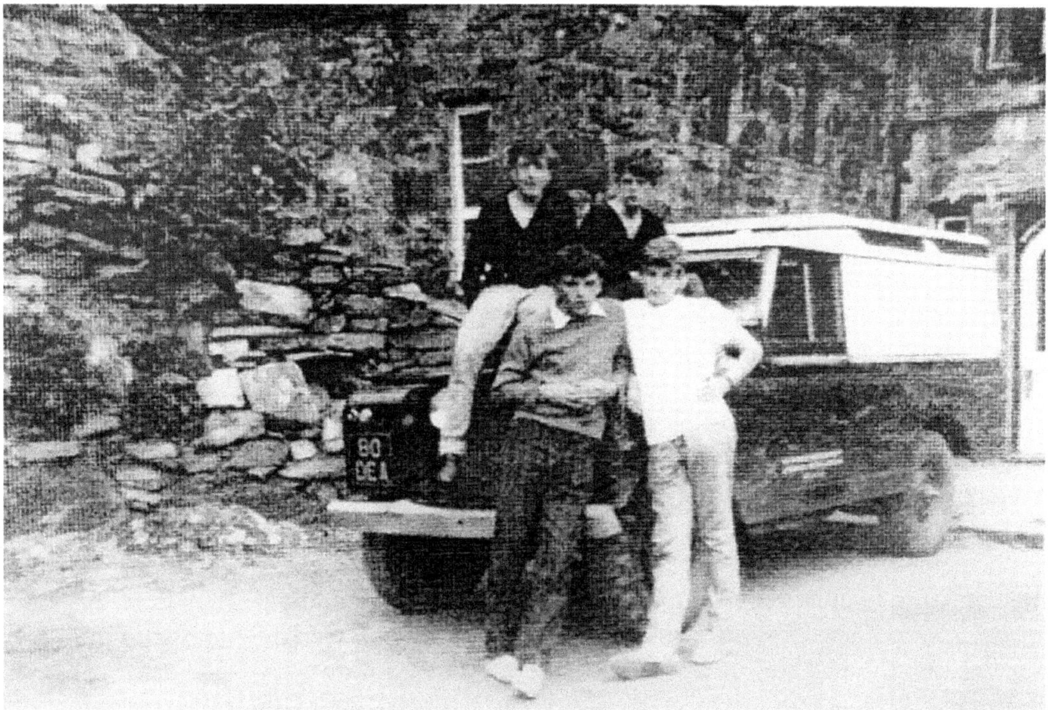

Top left Derrick Lees, top right David Holloway, front left Graham Collett, front right Patrick Edwards – all from George Salter School

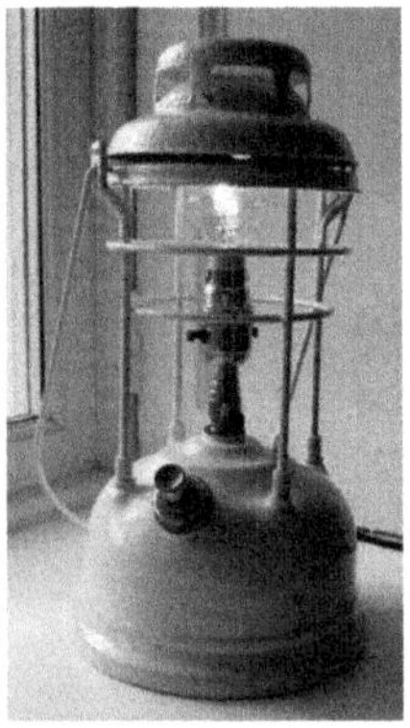

1950s Tilley Lamp

When I visited Plas there was no electricity. The daily chore was to clean and refill the Tilley lamps ready for the evening. Then there was the outside cold-water tap, situated approximately where the office and drying room is now. The outside wall by the original front door was used for practicing our rock-climbing skills, resulting in a few sprained ankles in the process when we fell off.

(Derrick continues to attend the annual reunions for those who attended during the 1950s, 60s and 70s).

Reg Snell shares his memories of Plas Gwynant 1962

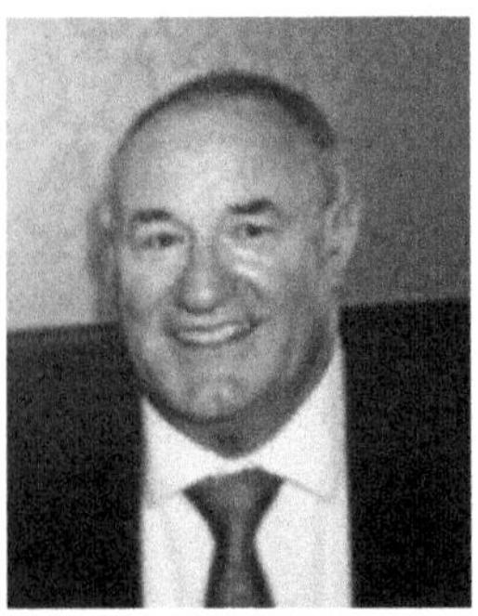

I started at Churchfields in 1958 and I was in Moore House. I went to Plas Gwynant I think it was in 1962, in which case I was in the fourth year and we stayed in tents in the fields below the house. I do remember that the cost was 15 shillings and that would have included the transport and food while we away. I seem to recall we were away for a week. But how we travelled there and how long we were really there, I can't remember.

The tents were ridge tents which held about six of us and there must have been 4 or 5 of these light green Niger tents, which suggests there could have been up to 30 of us. We did, daily, have to roll up the sides of the tents and move the groundsheets to prevent the grass from becoming damaged. Any other chores or duties that we had to do I simply cannot bring to mind. Whatever we did for washing and storing what clothes we brought I have no idea. I am sure to a fourteen or fifteen-year-old boy, washing was not that important!

On one occasion, we followed the Watkin Path and climbed up to the summit of Snowdon. We certainly had the minimum of correct equipment and appropriate clothing. We didn't have walking boots or socks. Who was in the party? (I will need help with this as I moved to Aldridge in my last year and lost touch with many of the people at school.). Names I can recall who went, who I have not seen since 1963 include in my year Robert Smith and Ian Williams. In the years above mine, David Spires (Spike) and Terry Simpson. Terry and Spike may have been staying in the house and helped us with climb to the summit. There were also younger pupils from the third year. The climb up was tiring but we achieved it without mishap.

We did go up the Watkin path again, later in the week.

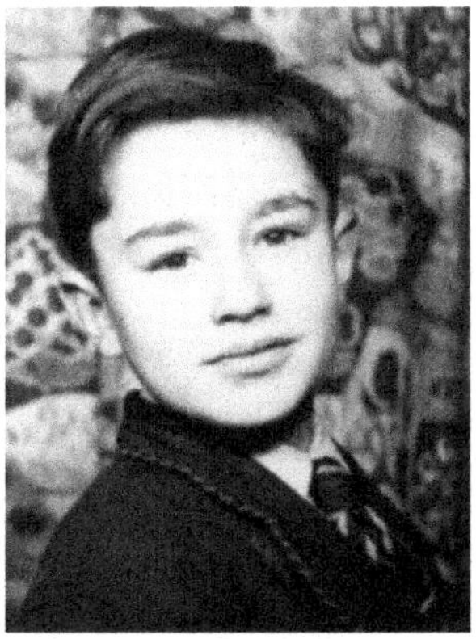

The plan, if there was one, was to camp overnight and do the summit again. About 10 of us took two or three small tents and got up near to the Gladstone rock where we set up camp. There was a teacher with us to look after us. Sadly, I cannot remember his name. I was in a tent with Spike, which we pitched and because of the wind anchored down the sides with rocks. We had some food and milk. Alongside was a gentle stream into which we placed the milk bottles to keep them cool. We were not daft! We would have fresh milk in the morning or so we thought.

It then started nonstop raining and pouring down. The other tents simply blew away and everyone was drenched. The teacher decided at around midnight that it would be safer to go back with the other youngsters, leaving Spike and me to look after ourselves, as we were relatively dry and safe. We did manage to sleep through the rest of the storm, waking to a dry morning. We then set to, making tea as we felt we had earned it after surviving the stormy night. Not for us, throwing in the towel as soon as it rained! We then had our comeuppance. The gentle stream of course, with all the rainfall, was now a raging torrent and about two feet higher than when we had stored the milk. Of which there was now no sight. There was no alternative, but to head back down the Watkin path to the camp and abandon our second climb up the summit.

An interesting experience, I think I enjoyed the week although now, over 55 years later, it seems like a faded dream in another world.

Derek Poulton - My reflections of a month spent at Plas Gwynant 1965

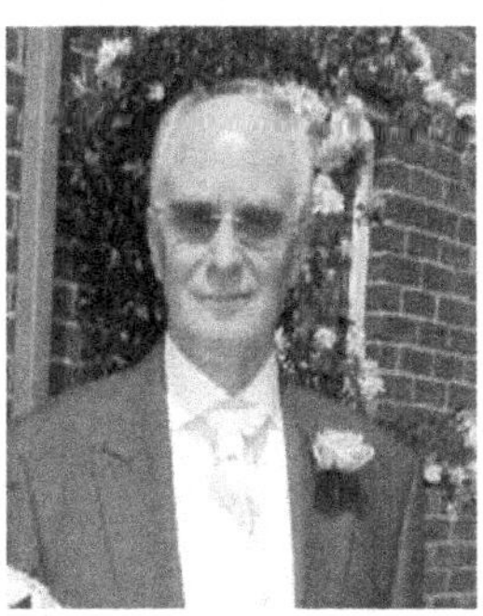

I spent a month at Plas Gwynant in July/August 1965, it has been 52 years so you can imagine due to time my memory is not too good at remembering any names, although I remember some events that happened quite well. Others who read this and were there at the same time as I was may be able to fill in the missing bits. I will attempt to put down on paper what I remember.

I had left Churchfields Comprehensive in July 1964, then aged 16, not having done well in exams due to my inability to understand at the time that an education was so important. I obtained a place at Brockhouse who were based at Hill Top West Bromwich as an apprentice, in those days they took anyone on. I believe about May 1965 I was asked by the apprentice department if I would like to go for a month on an 'Outward Bound' to Plas Gwynant. Some of the other apprentices were offered places at various similar outward bounds in different parts of the country. I jumped at the chance 4 weeks off work and another 2 weeks normal holiday when I returned because the factory was closed down for 2 weeks annual holiday, this sounded good.

I had the list of things I needed for the month and most important was a pair of strong mountain walking boots. I remember going into Birmingham city and buying a pair, they were all leather, not the greatest in comfort, but I was advised by the store assistant that they would gradually 'break in'. I don't remember where the group who were going to Plas Gwynant was picked up from, but I have a feeling it may have been outside the memorial gardens opposite the college in West Bromwich. I remember the coach journey both to and from Wales, this is because the driver was totally mad, music blaring and his driving was dire, how we got there and back in one piece is quite amazing, especially going around the mountainside roads in Wales. My mom had packed me off with sandwiches for the journey and I did not eat them, the coach parked on the road opposite the entrance to Plas Gwynant and the first thing I did was to chuck them away into a hedge, not good I know. The group had a large number of Churchfield pupils, mostly those I already knew from my time at School. Of the leaders, one was an ex Churchfield teacher, Mr Watterson he taught me maths and also PE, and one young leader was a very experienced climber. After settling in we were taken to the 'kit shed' and were issued with walking gear, I was over the moon with the quality of the anorak it was something I always remember, orange/red colour and I was reluctant to have to hand it back when we left.

On rising in the mornings, we were given the choice of a cross country run or a stroll down to the river where we were to take a dip. It was awfully cold and one morning we went down for a dip in the river but we decided it was too cold and just pretended we had done it. Yes, we got caught out and got a telling off. I decided in future to have the run rather the freeze to death in the river. During our time there we did various activities which included canoeing and rock climbing. The plan over the 4 weeks was to gradually build us up physically and give us the know-how to survive outdoors; sending us on expeditions with map references where there were tins to open and retrieve a code word, to prove we had been there. Gradually they got longer expeditions with the ultimate aim in the final week to send us on an overnight one.

We went on various expeditions as a group; on the first one they left us to decide what we took with us in our rucksacks, I remember taking my transistor radio as one item, we had to put together our rations which was dried food and it was not very appetising. After about a week we were put into groups of 4 and I think there was one group with 5 mainly 2 of each sex and a leader for each group was also chosen. We walked down the road in the direction of Pen y Pass and we climbed/ walked up alongside a large water pipe, some of you might know where it was exactly, possibly near Llyn Gwynant, the path is near Llyn Teyrn. It was tough going and most of us felt the strain of carrying too much weight, we learned the hard way and future expeditions we cut down to the minimum we needed to carry. Another expedition we went on we were supposed to go off road walk over a 'mountain' to where we were staying, a house in Capel Curig. When we got to the path to go off road, the visibility was poor it was lashing down with rain and we made a group decision for safety reasons to not go and walked to our destination along the road. When we arrived, and explained what we had done we got verbal lashing - we were not in the teachers' good books.

At Plas Gwynant there was always a school camp of a West Bromwich school that changed each week. One evening the boys plus teachers played the Grammar School, it was a blood and thunder football match, no prisoners taken and I got a nasty sprained ankle. Next morning, we were off to visit a copper mine, it was probably Sygun Copper Mine, not very commercialised at the time. I was struggling walking due to my football injuries and was one of the last to enter the mine. There was panic as one of the pupils had fallen 100 feet or so down the mine shaft – the young leader immediately abseiled down the shaft to him. He was unconscious but alive. Rescue gear was rushed to us, he was put on a stretcher and we after some hard work, all of us working together pulled him to the surface and carried him down to a waiting ambulance, where we were met by the mountain rescue team. We declined their help; we felt they were trying to get some credit for the rescue. It was an item of news in the local newspaper. He spent a few days in Bangor hospital, fortunately making a full recovery. I went to see him at his home when I got back, I don't remember his name but he lived at either Lilac Avenue or Almond Avenue Yew Tree Estate.

We climbed Snowdon via the Horseshoe, which was dangerous but the scenery was outstanding and it was brilliant weather so the views were clear. Sundays was a day off for the staff, so some of us we went off thumbing lifts to various places, Porthmadog and Beddgelert. The final expedition on the last week was upon us. We were kitted up with enough supplies for an overnight camp and tenting equipment. Each of the groups was dropped off at various locations and the aim was to be the first group to visit all the map locations and make it back to Plas Gwynant. My group was dropped off at Beddgelert and we made our way near Moel Y Dyniewyd heading towards Pen Y Gwryd where we set up camp had a meal and went for a lemon and lime in the Gwastadnant Hotel. All the groups were checked by a leader to make sure we were all well, he eventually found our group having difficulty in finding us because we had gone a lot further than he had anticipated no mobiles those days.

Next morning, we were up at the crack of dawn and off to find the next grid reference which was near Llyn Teyrn, we went via Pen y Pass. We were so far advanced that we caught up with the group who had camped next to Llyn Teyrn and from there we went together with the other group. It took a toll on us and I was flagging, so to save time I remember the last grid reference we had to find a few of us had a rest and the fitter of the 2 groups went and found it.

We made our way back to Plas Gwynant and the other group still had another grid reference to find but they threw the towel in and also came back with us. They later regretted this because their failure to complete the expedition meant that when it was discovered, they got a severe verbal bashing.

Overall the best 4 weeks holiday I have ever had - seems like yesterday, not 52 years ago.

Plas Gwynant House

Following the connection to electricity in 1966 and the installation of proper sewage disposal in 1967, the house became habitable for students, dispensing with the need for tents within the grounds – though some have expressed sadness at losing the camping.
The early photographs show a much smaller facility than the modern, extended one of today, though the charm of the building is retained.

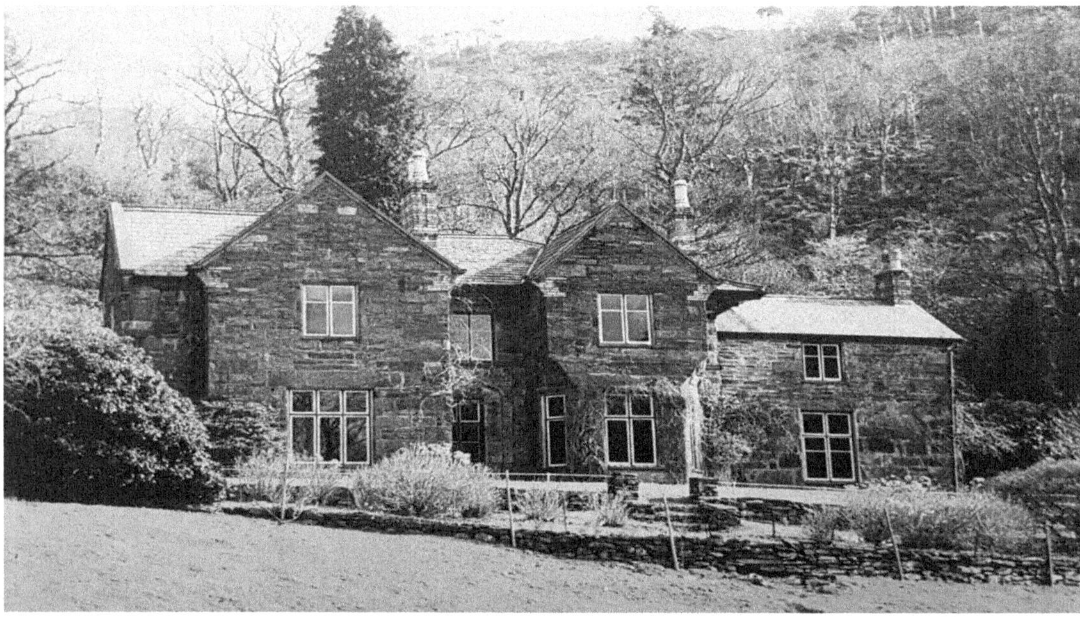

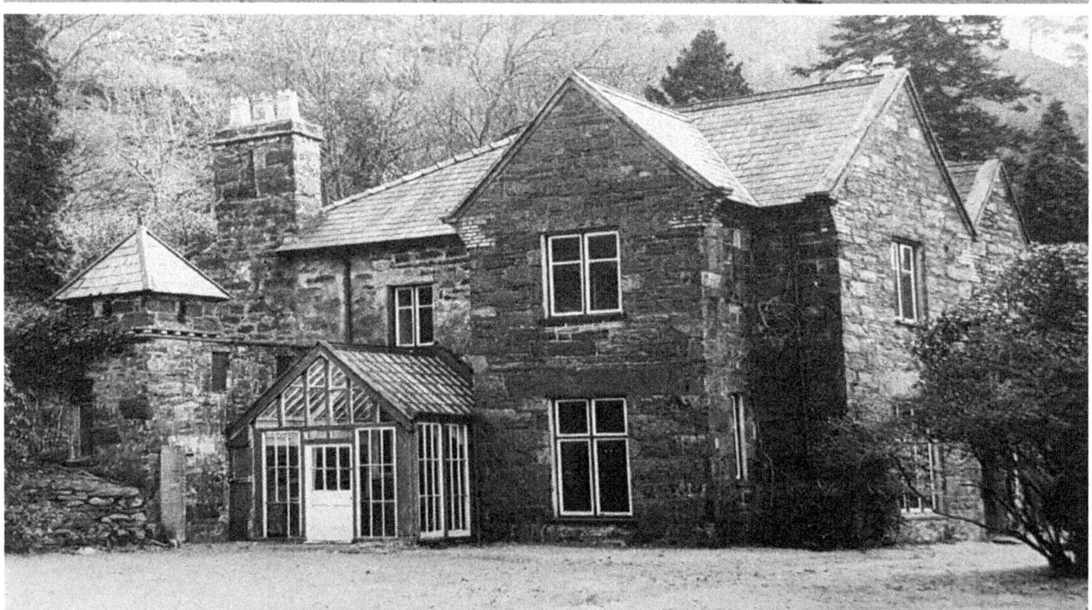

Stephen Edwards shares his memories of Plas Gwynant 1965

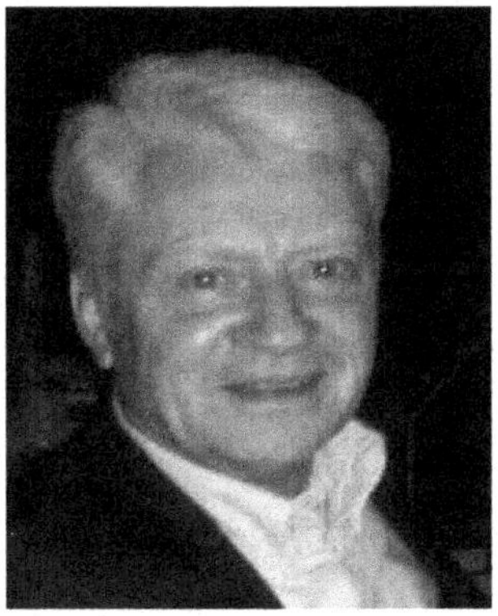

I was very fortunate to go to Plas Gwynant in January 1965.
I went to Spon Lane Secondary Modern School, and at the time Mr Watterson was our deputy headmaster. I think he had a lot to do with us having the opportunity to go to Plas Gwynant.

It was a wonderful experience and, although being in the middle of winter, it was one of the best things that ever happened to me during my school days.

I remember that it was really cold and, one morning near the beginning of the course, when Scottie Dwyer woke us up for the mandatory shower, none of us were keen to get up. We all stayed in bed until we heard Scotty coming back up the stairs, when we jumped out and all said that we'd already had our showers. He said that he found that quite strange, as the showers were still dry! He then ordered us to strip off and stand in a line by the showers, and one by one he held us by our necks under the cold water. We learnt our lesson, and didn't do it again.

One very memorable occasion was 24th January, the day when Winston Churchill died. We were ordered down to the assembly room, where a long speech was given about this great man. I remember at the time thinking that he really couldn't have been that great as he was not a member of the Labour Party!

There were many occasions and incidents that made my stay at Plas Gwynant so special and such a positive influence on my life, but one occasion really stands out and has remained with me ever since. We were all given a chore to do. I can no longer remember what mine was, but a friend, Philip Whiston, was given the task of cleaning the outside toilet. Of course, we all made fun of him, and kept reminding him that he was the toilet cleaner. No doubt we were all happy not to have to do that particular job!

On the final day of the course we had a farewell meeting. Everyone was praised for their part and for the effort all had put in to make the course a success. At the end of the speeches, the head of the Centre said that he wanted to praise one person in particular for his contribution. Everyone else was no doubt thinking ' it must be me!' Of course, it was none other than Philip Whiston, for cleaning the toilet! Despite all the stick he had taken from us, he ended up the hero. He had in fact done a wonderful job of a not particularly nice task, and the toilet, throughout our stay, was immaculate. I had learnt an important life lesson - it's not what you do but how you do it that is the most important.

Olwyn Bailey (nee Edwards) shares her memories of Plas Gwynant

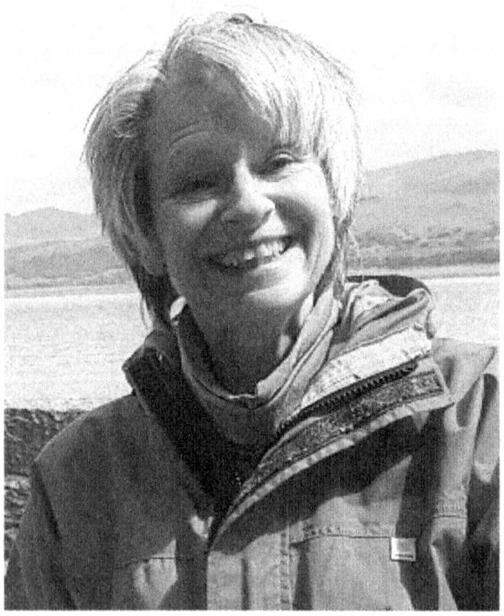

I count myself very fortunate to have had the opportunity to stay at Plas Gwynant a few times in my teenage years, either on Geography or Biology field trips. All my memories of those visits are happy, and of a time spent with good friends in the most beautiful place. We would get on the coach in the industrial air of West Bromwich and get off to the smell of the pure air of Snowdonia.

On one occasion, we were dropped off in groups of three, with a map, somewhere fairly remote from which point we had to make our way back to Plas Gwynant. Our group managed to walk to Beddgelert, where we bought an ice-cream and pondered the remainder of the long walk back to base. Surely, there was nothing to stop us thumbing a lift to save ourselves the trouble of walking? This we did, and quickly got a lift from a local farmer in his Land Rover. He dropped us by the gate, and we took our time walking up the drive (not wanting to appear too early).

When we arrived, the staff seemed inexplicably unhappy with us. We expected them to be impressed at how quickly we had navigated our way back, but instead we were lectured on the folly of three young girls thumbing a lift with a stranger. The farmer had telephoned the centre and dobbed us in!

Most nights, well after lights out, we arranged to meet our friends for a 'midnight feast', which involved jumping out of the upstairs dorm window onto a grassy bank, and walking round to the old drying room. The most difficult part was the return journey, sneaking past the staff bedrooms, but we never got caught.

Fine mornings were always started with a pre-breakfast dip in the river - something else not strictly allowed. I seem to mostly recall all the things I shouldn't have been doing, but I do still remember some geographical and ecological facts gleaned along the way, so perhaps it wasn't a complete waste of education.

What has remained with me, more than anything, is a deep and abiding love of North Wales. As an adult, I return at least twice a year, and never fail to remember, and feel grateful for, those times I spent at Plas Gwynant.

Lynn Woodward (nee Edwards) shares her memories

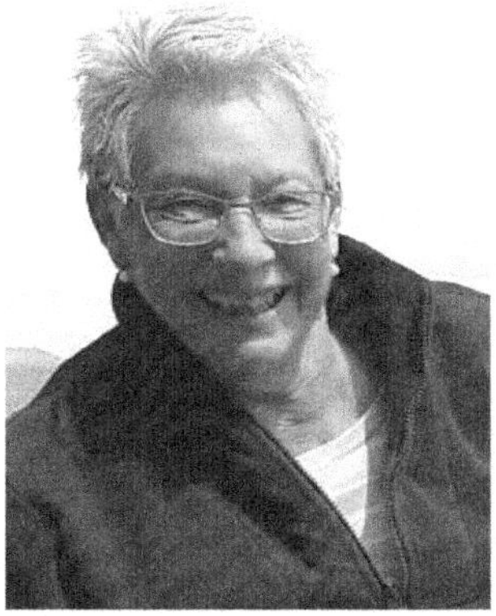

I attended Churchfields Comprehensive School between 1959 and 1964 but although I desperately wanted to go to Plas Gwynant I was never given the opportunity, much to my disappointment, which was made worse when my brother and sister both younger than me were able to go!

When my sister saw on Facebook about the reunion weekends and suggested we go, I jumped at the chance. The nearest I had got before was camping in a field nearby.

Although I didn't know anyone because of our similar ages and going to the same schools I found the atmosphere brilliant. It was great to be able to take part in the activities and push myself to do more than I would have thought, although I still do not like heights.

It was also nice to have modern facilities now like electricity - I have heard lots about Tilley Lamps! A fabulous weekend which I look forward to now every year and in fact have already booked for next year.

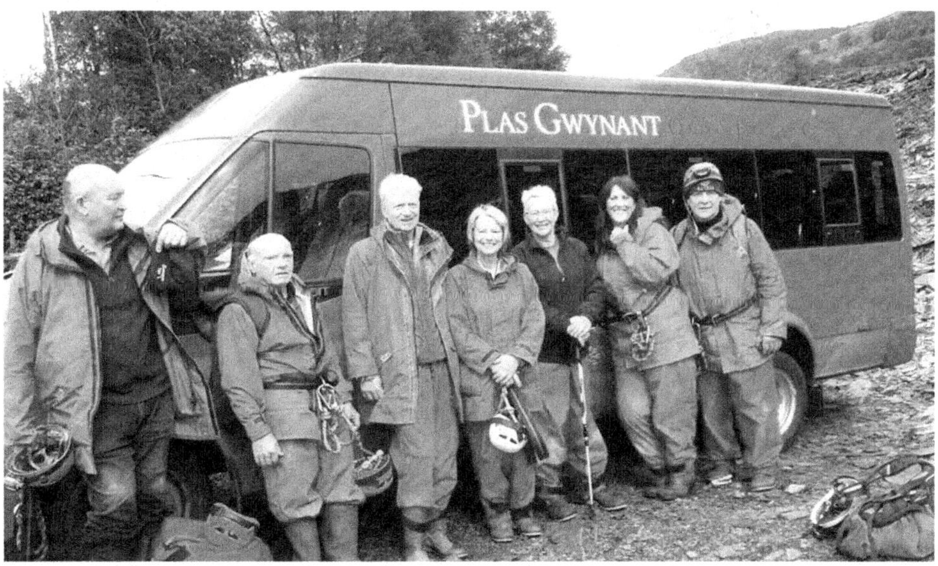

2016 Reunion: Roy Simms, Wally Gough, Steven Edwards, Olwyn Bailey, Lynn Woodward, Jan Drury and Frank Batchelor

(The 'Edwards siblings', Steven, Olwyn and Lynn, continue to attend the annual Plas Gwynant Reunions for those who attended in the 1950's, 60's and 70's, as do the others in the photograph).

Memories from Gary Rushton

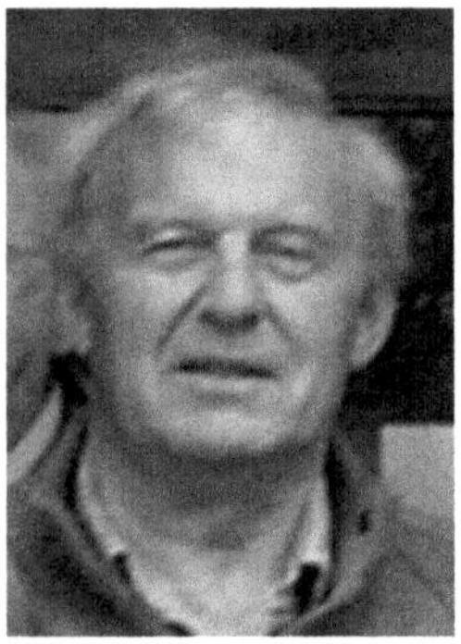

Gary has provided an in-depth personal account of his ongoing experiences at Plas Gwynant, which began in 1960. Gary writes:
When I first arrived in West Bromwich in the harsh winter of 1947, I was just six weeks old. At first my parents took care of me in the front room of my grandparents' home in Law Street, on the Tantany Estate. Later we moved to an old condemned terraced house in Cophall Street, Great Bridge, but in 1952 a newly built council house on Yew Tree Estate came our way. It was from there that I went to Churchfields Comprehensive School in 1958, when this showpiece establishment was just three years old. My first two years at Churchfields were not happy ones. However, nothing lasts forever, and circumstances took a turn for the better in 1960.

Back then, during the summer months, secondary schools in West Bromwich were able to send groups of boys (and separate groups of girls I think) to a camp in North Wales. I believe that initially this facility had been set up in the Beddgelert forest but when Plas Gwynant was acquired in the late 1950s, the camp was relocated to the field in front of the main house. I was first persuaded to go on a weeks' camp by my friends Desmond Dawes and Peter Reynolds, who I believe had some background in this activity as scouts or Boys Brigade. I will be forever grateful to them both.

Each school group was transported to the camp by coach and stayed for a week, Friday to Friday as I recall. The coach would then return to deliver a new group and take those thirty or so exhausted and somewhat soiled individuals, and their accompanying teachers, back to West Bromwich. My parents paid the required fifteen shillings (75p) and acquired for me a sleeping bag which, together with a waterproof bicycle cape, plate, mug and KFS, (knife, fork and spoon) was all the equipment needed. On the day everything was packed into an old kit bag and stowed in the boot of the coach, together with a couple of boys' pushbikes and off we went. The bikes enabled us to pick up the odd groceries from Beddgelert. The infrastructure of the camp was what might be best described as 'heavy' or 'static' and consisted of the following:

- Six-man ridge tents (five or six in number I recall)
- A large marquee tent with wooden benches and tables for dining, etc.
- A smaller tent which functioned as a larder / food store
- A cook tent (roof sheet only) provided with a wood fired iron hot plate and oven arrangement (no bottled gas here!)

Everything described above was cotton canvas, either white, pale green or khaki coloured. Guy ropes were hemp and poles and pegs were wooden – modern materials were nowhere to be seen. It all had a distinctive smell, especially when damp, which was pretty much all of the time! Fresh water was obtained several times each day from a tap located near the main house and transported in what can be best described as a galvanised dustbin on wheels. Elsan-type toilets were located in the old stable block, in what is now the store room for jackets and over-trousers. Despite my ability to recall much of the camp layout, it seems that I have chosen to wipe away any memory of how the contents of these facilities were disposed of. Neither can I remember how we washed ourselves, if indeed we did.

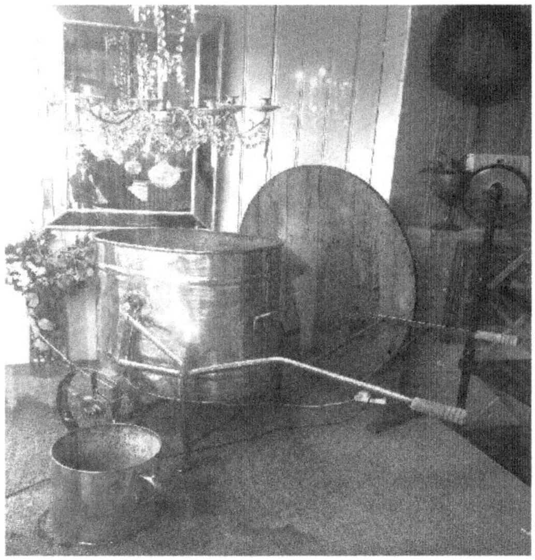

Above: A 'galvanised dustbin' - this contraption seen recently in the window of an antique shop in Sussex is practically identical in size, shape and form to the one used at school camps in the 1960s.

We were of course accompanied by two or three of our teachers who had volunteered to supervise us for the week. There was no interplay as I recall between us campers and the staff at Plas Gwynant. In fact, on that first 1960 visit I don't think that I was even aware of the name Plas Gwynant. To me it was simply school camp in Snowdonia. I can recall the names of two of the teachers who accompanied us on that first trip. One was Mr Fathers, who taught geography and the other was the aptly named, Mr Camplin. 'Daddy' Fathers was a great bloke for this sort of activity. He knew how to channel the energy of a group of young boys in a positive, wholesome and fun way. I remember well the water fights we had with him and the wrestling free-for-alls. I also remember he took us up Snowdon via the Watkin Path on a beautiful summer day. In the following year we did Tryfan after a bus ride up to the Pen-y-Gwryd and, in my third and final camp (summer 1962) Mr Fathers took three of us up to Gladstone Rock for an overnight camp. For this 'high camp' experience we used some of Churchfields lightweight camping equipment that the school had acquired for Duke of Edinburgh purposes. There was another good guy called Mr Page (can't recall his subject) as well as Fred Luke the PE teacher. I never found Mr Luke to be very approachable, but I'm sure that he had his fans.

The experience of school camp, particularly that first one in 1960, made me realise that some of the teachers at Churchfields were in fact quite normal people who could conduct themselves in ways that I could respond to.

Layout of the grounds at Plas Gwynant showing the Location of some of its main features

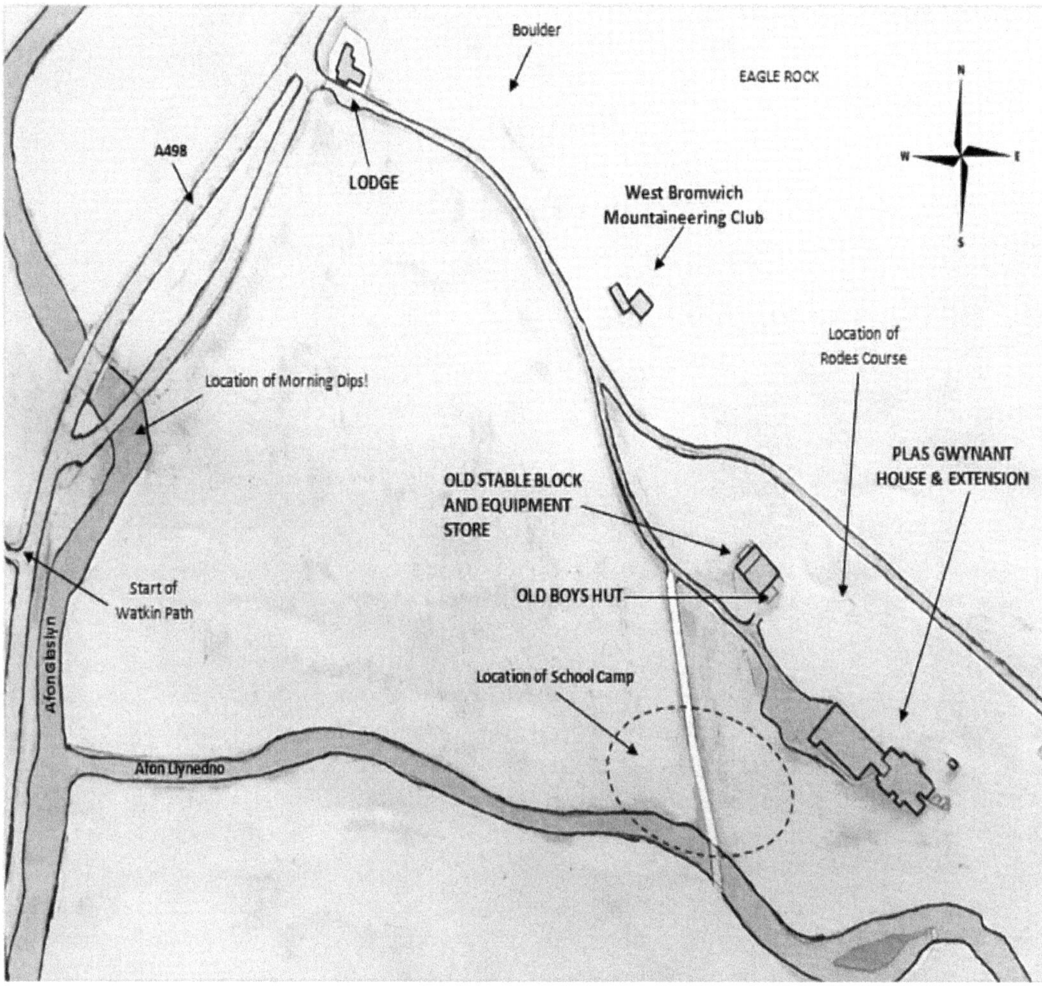

That first school camp may have been my first real experience of teamwork. The camp was organised in such a way that each day one tent (of four, five or six boys) was responsible for cooking, washing up, fire duties, etc. It was all great fun and there was a tremendous element of adventure and freedom. This, together with the experience of being away from home for the first time, seemed to have a profound effect on me and my relationship with school. From the start of the third year I recall being much happier, more confident and very much more in tune with school life.

School camp had another profound effect on me, one which is perhaps difficult to appreciate in this day and age. Britain in the early 1960s was emerging from a period of grey, monotonous austerity (where austerity meant exactly that) and was entering an era where, amongst other things, travel, communication, colour and choice would be plentiful. And, like many of my contemporaries, up to that point in time I had barely set foot outside of the West Midlands conurbation. So imagine my surprise when, in 1960 I was greeted by beautiful mountains, jagged ridges, steep hillsides with crags and boulders, crystal-clear streams and noisy waterfalls. Compared to West Bromwich, everything before me seemed clean and fresh. I think I knew, there and then, that I had to keep returning to these surroundings, however long or short my life would be. Without hesitation therefore, I signed up for a second school camp in 1961, this time persuading my friend Roger Freeman to come along and again in the summer of 1962. I didn't do the 1963 camp because it clashed with a month-long stay at Plas Gwynant proper. And by 1964 or 65, school camps at Plas were no longer being offered to West Bromwich school children. A sad loss!

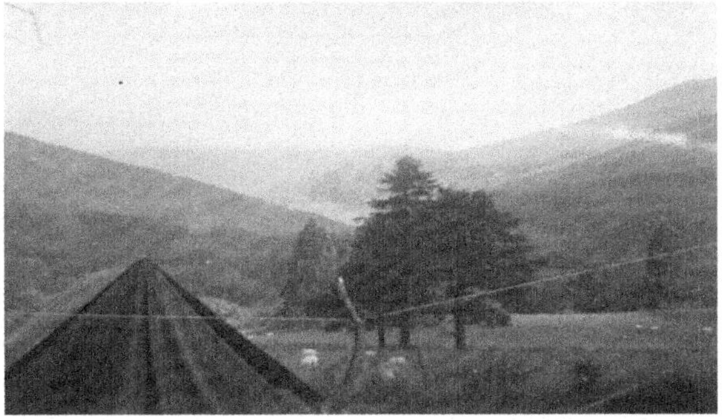

The food store tent, school camp 1960

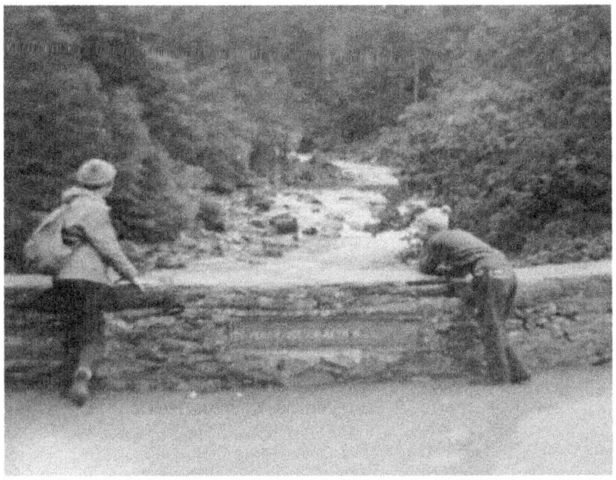

Gary Rushton and Desmond Dawes contemplating the wonders of Aberglaslyn 1960

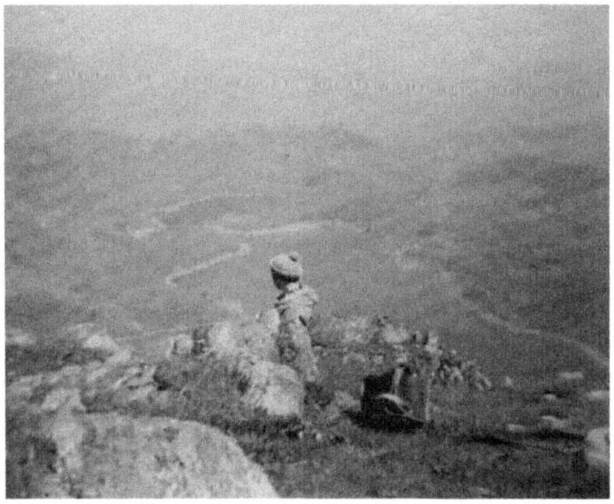

Gary Rushton looking at Llyn Llydau from the ridge between Snowdon and Lliwedd (Bwlch y Saethau) 1961

Back in the early 1960s, month-long courses were the core business of Plas and because I had enjoyed school camp so much, I had no hesitation in taking up this opportunity. The experience began on Monday 2 April 1962 when the coach left Highfields in Carters Green. This lovely building was then the offices of West Bromwich Education Department and the place where Mr Turner (Director of Education) and Bert Wright (Head of Physical Activities) would have been based. It was these two individuals I believe who were responsible for setting up Plas Gwynant and for giving the boys and girls of the borough the golden opportunities that it provided.

Before describing the activities and the advantages that were on offer at Plas, it is worth pointing out one detail that I suspect has been long forgotten in the years between now and then. At the bottom of the driveway leading up to Plas, close to the Lodge, there was a sign board, much as there is today. However, unlike those that followed it, the original that I can still picture in my mind was bold in form and told new arrivals exactly what to expect: PLAS GWYNANT ADVENTURE SCHOOL – and adventure was what you got.

The courses at Plas Gwynant were 26 days long and arranged on the Outward Bound principle. Boys and girls were taught a variety of outdoor skills, such as map reading and compass work, lightweight camping practice and survival in mountain terrain, rock climbing and abseiling, canoeing, first aid, estate work and ropes course. Participants were divided up from day one into groups of about five or six (patrols with names such as Hebog, Tryfan or Ogwen), thereby ensuring that teamwork was an important underlying theme. That said, I believe that each boy or girl who attended the course was given every opportunity to blossom individually and develop to the best of their ability. And it was this attribute that made Plas Gwynant so very special in those early years. I was lucky enough to take part in three of these courses involving a total of about 60 boys and I don't recall any one of them leaving at the end of the stay with doubts about their accomplishments. Without exception it seemed to me that everyone experienced a gain in self-confidence as a result of their experiences at Plas and the activities undertaken. Badges were given out at the end of the course and were received with great pride.

Those who were lucky enough to be there will remember some of the lesser activities I am sure. I know that this is how it is for me. For example, back in the early 1960s, there was no mains electricity in the valley. Everyone who was there at that time will remember the ritual of lighting the Tilley lamps when darkness fell on the house. And who can forget running down to the river Glaslyn at 6.30 each morning for a dip in the icy cold water. And what about the indoor sports undertaken in the common room (now part of the dining room), or the challenge of unprepared public speaking on a topic allotted to you just ten seconds beforehand! I remember there weren't many occasions when you were given time to feel homesick.

I'm not sure if it is the same nowadays but back then the school day had to begin with an assembly and some sort of obligatory religious lesson, and so it was at Plas Gwynant, (when you weren't waking up in a tent on some wet hillside). However, what I found refreshingly different was that the lessons there were taken from newspaper cuttings (or similar) and were usually about everyday people and events. They were easier to relate to, unlike those taken from the scriptures. I recall the one about a seven-stone American woman who, when her husband became trapped beneath a car he had been working on, had summoned the strength to lift it and pull him out safely.

It was also in the common room that I first discovered the joys of folk music. One of the instructors had a wind-up or battery operated gramophone and a small collection of LP records by Pete Seeger and Joan Baez.

A description of life at Plas Gwynant would not be complete without mentioning the contributions made by the various staff members. Most important of all was George Simpkin, who we knew as the Warden (no wonder some of my contemporaries at school were filled with dread at the prospect of a month-long stay at this place!) For me, George Simpkin is the forgotten hero and deserves much more credit than he has since received from some quarters. My understanding was that he had previously worked for the Outward Bound Trust at Eskdale in the Lake District and, in an earlier life, had walked all the way around Tasmania. He was, I am convinced the person most responsible for giving Plas its 'structure' and for seeding those wonderful memories that many of us now have. He was a gentle man with a young family. It seemed to me that he had the respect of everyone around him and he didn't need to raise his voice to gain that respect. Intuitively he seemed to strike the right balance between discipline, guidance, encouragement and hard work that enabled boys and girls to develop into confident young adults. I remember that he liked the works of Rudyard Kipling and, presumably Lewis Carroll because, on the long day exercise, many of the hidden tins that we were searching out contained clue words, such as brillig, slithy, tove, etc.

On the first course that I attended in 1962, George was assisted by three instructors: George (Scotty) Dwyer, Terry Parker and Paul Hill. Scotty Dwyer was an old man of the mountains. He walked with a limp due to a hip problem, possibly arthritis or similar, and I remember feeling quite sorry for him as he tackled some steep slopes with a sack on his back. I never heard him complain. I remember he was still working at Plas in 1965 after Parker and Hill had moved on. Terry Parker was tall and lean, that's about all I can remember apart from the fact that he took Ozzie Brookes and myself up a climb called Reineta at Tremadoc and suffered what I can best describe as a 'melt-down'. Paul Hill had worked as a journalist for the Express and Star newspaper in Wolverhampton. I met him some years later at his home near Brassington in Derbyshire where he was running photographic courses.

My diary also records several other members of staff. There was Miss Wilson (housekeeper) and Miss Pritchat (cook). I have her to thank for all the tasty food I received and for her patience in teaching me how to say that long place name in Anglesey (you know the one: Llanfairpwllgwyngyllgogerychwyrndrobwllllantysiliogogogoch). And I wouldn't want to forget the warden's two dogs, Kipling and Kayla. Kipling did the Snowdon Horseshoe with us towards the end of the course and I have to say his traverse of Crib Goch was a good deal more stylish than mine.

The cost to parents for a month at Plas Gwynant was initially £3.50 but I think this was later increased to £5. In my school we paid the money over to Mr Watterson, who also dealt with the application forms, etc. However, despite this ridiculously small sum of money, there were times when it had not been possible to fill the twenty odd places on the course, especially in the winter. In part this must have been due to the size of the catchment, (remember this was West Bromwich and not Sandwell). But other factors such as the course's reputation for difficult and uncomfortable activities, its perceived similarities with National Service and simple apathy were also at play I suspect. On more than one occasion in my school I can recall overhearing some loudmouth, bully-boy type proclaim that he wouldn't be going to Plas Gwynant because it was too demanding and involved too much discomfort! Such utterances gave me quiet satisfaction.

Courses that were not fully subscribed must have disappointed some (the Director of Education for example). But from my point of view it was good news because it gave me and some of my friends the opportunity to sign up for a second stint of adventure.

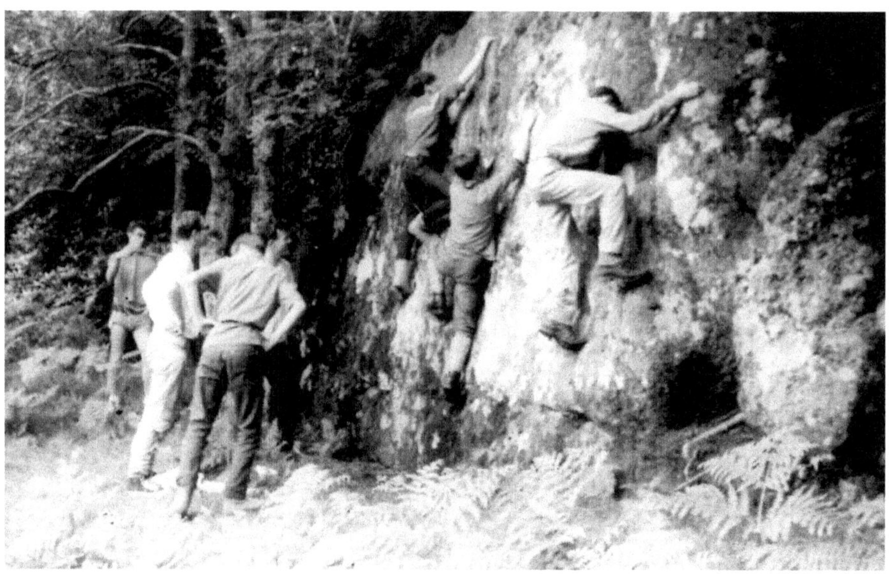

The 1963 Course - Boulder climbing at the rear of Plas Gwynant Lodge
Standing: Roger Freeman, Ray Durden, Gary Rushton. Climbing: Pete Johnson, Ron Wood and Trevor Clarke. (The person standing at the rear may be V McCormack)

The 15 July 1963 saw me depart from Highfields yet again and, from diaries that we were obliged to keep at the time, I can see that this second course involved a similar range of activities to the previous year. However, many of the routes and locations were different. Also, the weather was better and the days longer, so the overall impression (and the reality) was that this 26-day course was tougher and more arduous than the one a year earlier. Added to this was the fact that a few bigger boys were included – apprentices rather than schoolboys. For me this made the whole experience a lot more enjoyable because we were 'stretched' to the limit at times. For example, I well remember the Carneddau expedition where, towards the end of day one, three of the lads were so exhausted that we had to carry their rucksacks as well as our own before reaching our campsite near the tiny lake of Ffynnon Lloer at 9.30pm. Similarly, with the 'long day' scheme, a two-day expedition which involved approximately 40 miles, 9000 feet of ascent and 25 hours of walking. Oh, to be as fit as that now!

One of my enduring recollections was that when it was all over and I was back home, I met up with a friend who asked me what I thought about the daring robbery that had taken place a few days earlier. "What robbery?" I replied. "The great Train Robbery" she answered. Difficult to imagine nowadays but back then in Nant Gwynant we were nicely cut off from the rest of the world.

How good that was!

I don't know how many youngsters in West Bromwich were given the opportunity to go on two courses at Plas Gwynant; besides myself, I know of at least six – Roger Bainbridge, Roger Freeman, Royston Simms, Peter Johnson, John Turton and Raymond Durden. However, I think Bainbridge, Freeman and myself must hold the record because we even managed a third, albeit shorter course, in January 1964.

This third excursion did not overlap with any school holidays, as the previous two had done. I remember that Mr Spinks (Head of Maths at Churchfields) was not at all impressed that Raymond Durden and I would be missing for two weeks of A-Level tuition! And if I'm truthful there were one or two occasions during that fortnight when I thought that I had made the wrong call and should have stuck with Mr Spinks. That's because those two weeks were very, very cold and wet, so much so that we were issued with two sleeping bags for our nights out under canvas – bivouac sheets, not tents!

Again, the course content was much the same as before, but necessarily condensed. There were two new members of staff by then; Alan Hole and Dave Yates. Dave was a very good rock climber. He took me, Bainbridge and Freeman up Crackstone Rib during that fortnight, my first rock climb in Llanberis Pass. Dave told us how he had lived in Kingstanding as a youth and used to hitch up to Wales starting from The Beggars Bush public house. He was the inspiration for later exploits by Bainbridge and me. Many years later I came across Dave and his wife Lilian, who he told me had been a housekeeper at Plas, although I could not recall her. They were running a chandlery shop in Victoria Harbour, Caernarvon.

On this winter course there were only eight or nine West Bromwich boys, the other participants were derived from a sixth form group at Marlborough Public School in Wiltshire. Obviously, a case of somebody being able to pull a few strings! Despite obvious differences in background (extreme in some cases), we all got on well together, but these lads were something else! Many didn't know how to wash up or make a cup of tea – and I'm not exaggerating! Needless to say, not one of them suffered from home-sickness but there were other health issues on this course. One Marlborough boy fell out of a tree which was part of the ropes course, fractured his jaw and had to be sent home on the train from Bangor. Another boy from West Bromwich suffered hypothermia whilst camping out near Pen-y-Gwryd. These issues aside, to me it is a testament to what outward bound courses of this type can achieve. At one end of the spectrum were boys from council houses where the family had only enough resources to get them through to the end of the week. At the other end were wealthy boys, some of whom were millionaires in waiting. Yet from the outset we all got on and worked well together. And if further proof of that were needed, it came some months later when we West Bromwich lads were invited by the Marlborough boys to stay at their school as their guests. We journeyed down there by coach and spent a long weekend with them, sleeping in their dormitories, joining in their lessons and their choir practice, etc., and eating with them in the free-for-all that was their dining arrangement. What an eye-opener that was! I have often wondered what happened to the Marlborough boys. Roger Bainbridge and I did make some attempts in 2011 to contact them as part of the 50-year Plas Anniversary, but we were not successful. It is also unfortunate that I do not have a group photograph for the 1964 course.

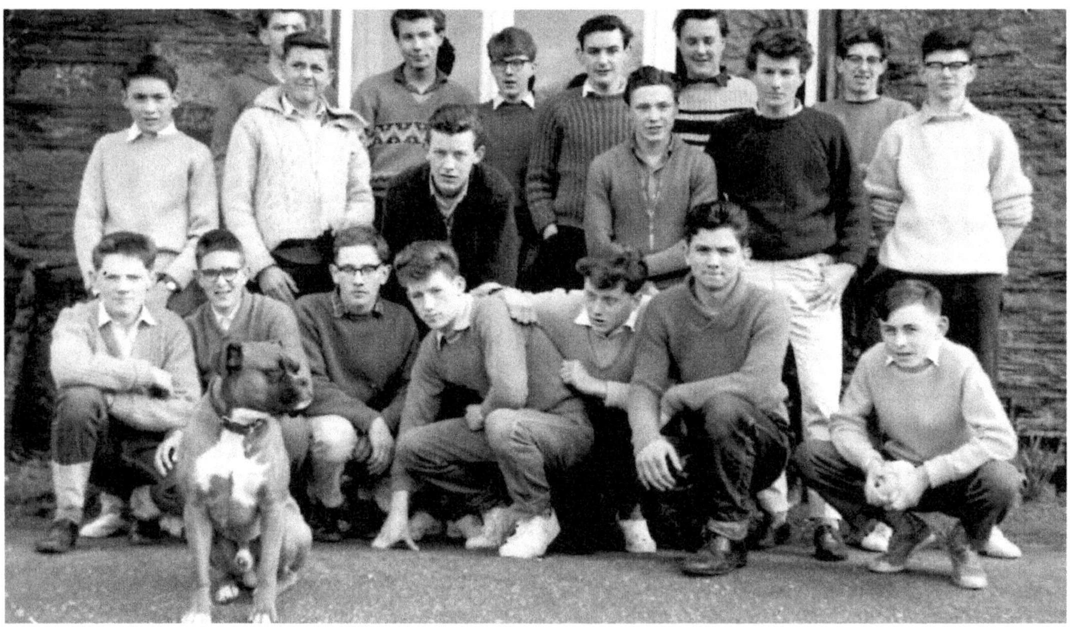

The 1962 Course - Back row, L-R: C Mellor, C Heal, Larry Brookes, John Turton, J Hutchings and G Davies Middle row L-R: Roy Simms, M Toon, Gary Rushton, D Edwards, N Jones and G Scullard. Front row L-R: P Johnson, Desmond Dawes, Roger Freeman, Dorian Dugmore, Robert Sadler, H Marshall and Roger Bainbridge. (Dog: Kipling)

I can't recall how I first learned that there was a facility by which boys and girls who had previously attended a 26-day course could return to Plas and stay there, free of charge. It was probably that trio of friends – Roy (Sid) Simms, Lawrence (Ozzy) Brookes and Pete Johnson who first brought the 'old Boys Hut' to the attention of me and my gang. Sometime in 1962/63 George Simpkin made available the lean-to building which forms the right hand side of the stable block where the equipment is now stored. His idea was that if you could find your way up to North Wales, you could have a roof over your head at no cost. Perhaps he felt that any charge would have been embarrassing given the very basic nature of the hut. It comprised very crude timber bunks (think of those grainy black and white images of Auschwitz), an old dining table and a broken chair / bed. A year on, an old iron stove from the drying room in Plas Gwynant was installed. It didn't work very well and on one occasion I remember returning home after a long stay, during which we used the stove almost continuously, in an effort to keep warm. My mother remarked that I smelled like a kipper.

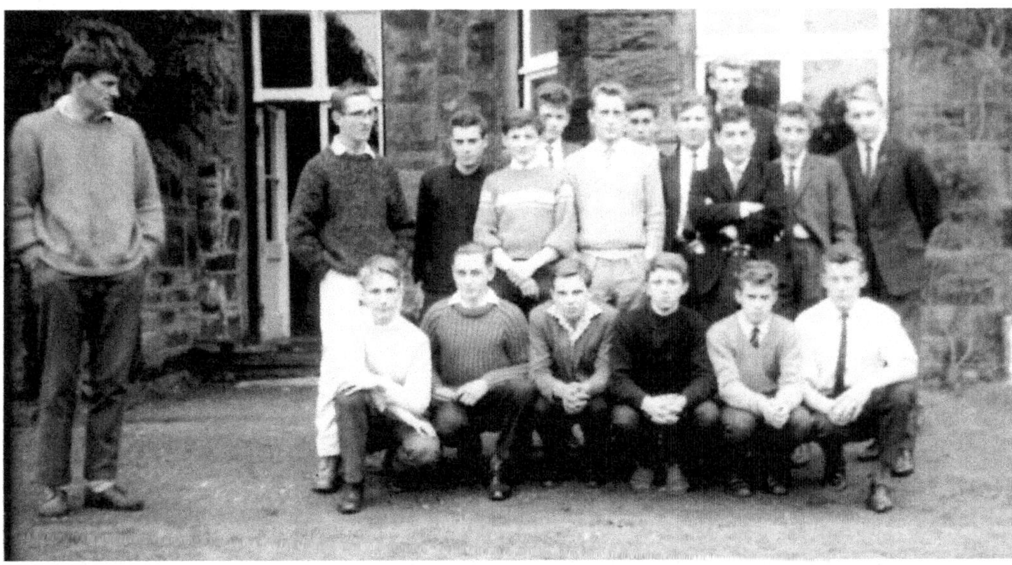

The 1963 Course - Back row, L-R: James Crowley, Roy Simms and Stan Fletcher. Middle row L-R: Roger Freeman, D Richards, Pete Johnson, Bob Parry, Dave Harper, Bob Gould, Ray Durden and Barry Jone. Front row L-R: Trevor Clarke, Roger Bainbridge, David Overton, Ron Wood, V McCormick and Gary Rushton. Standing at the far left is Terry Parker

I am told that there was no front wall on the hut in those early days but when I first reached there in May 1963 some additional protection in the form of a shed door, timber lower panel and polythene windows had been added. The floor space measured 12 feet by 8 feet or thereabouts, but it was perfect for a small group of young boys. No parents, no teachers, no running water and no electricity. Water had to be obtained in Billy-cans from the outside tap at the rear of the house. For lighting we used candles or an old coffee tin filled with paraffin and provided with a bootlace wick. Cooking was by means of a primus stove.

My first visit to the Old Boys Hut was in May 1963 with Alan (Whacka) Morris, Roger Bainbridge, Roger Freeman and Raymond Durden. Whacka and I made the journey on a tandem bicycle complete with pannier bags, rucksack and pup tent strapped to the crossbar. It took 13 hours from West Bromwich but we did it in one day and didn't need to use the tent. The others in the party took advantage, quite literally, of rail transport. My understanding is that the technique went something like this –
A fall guy was appointed. Supposedly he was in charge of looking after the tickets. When, and if, a ticket collector appeared, a great theatrical performance ensued. Said fall guy was berated by his accomplices for having lost the tickets. Act two involved spreading the contents of rucksacks across the seats of the carriage in an attempt to locate the 'missing' tickets. When eventually the ticket collector rumbled the plot and demanded payment, the grand finale ensued. During this time all three actors made their bids for Oscar nomination by pretending to have boarded at the last stop and to be no older than 13!

That five-night was the highlight of my life up to that point in time. The weather was marvellous, the friendship was wonderful and the nights were late. We climbed Lockwoods Chimney, ate lots of baked beans and did many miles of mountain walking. But it was the sense of freedom that I remember most. School camp three years earlier had been a great adventure for me, so too had my 26-day course in 1962, but this was something even better.

Throughout the second half of 1963 and 1964 we returned many times to the Old Boys Hut but by this stage we had all learned to use the thumb! Hitch-hiking was a wonderful way of getting around in those days and we weren't limited to North Wales. With the aforementioned friends, and others, I remember getting to the Lake District, The Scottish Highlands, Pontesford Rocks in Shropshire, Black Rock in Derbyshire, Devon and Cornwall and many other places. Only on a very few occasions did I have to spend the night sleeping under a hedge!

It was during this period that Bainbridge, Freeman and I joined the Wednesbury Climbing Club. Their mini bus provided another way of getting to Wales. It was also when Bainbridge and I did many of the difficult/severe classic rock climbs in the Llanberis and Ogwen areas. Routes such as Crevice, Sabre Cut, The Cracks and Tennis Shoe. From time to time we would vary our accommodation by staying in a barn situated below Ogwen falls or by sleeping under the Cromlech Boulders in Llanberis.

In the autumn of 1965 I went to university in London and I can't recall many visits to the Old Boys Hut during that first academic year. The focus seemed to be more on Ogwen at that time. However, towards the end of 1966 Roger Bainbridge and I made a purposeful decision to return to the Old Boys Hut and I invited along a university friend called Ron Canty. Ron was a very good rock climber and he took Bainbridge and myself up routes that we hadn't dare attempt before. A short time later, having realised the potential of the hut, the three of us undertook some improvement works. Scaffold planks and second-hand mattresses were brought up from London to improve sleeping arrangements and the hut was given a general tidy up.

The Brocken Spectre

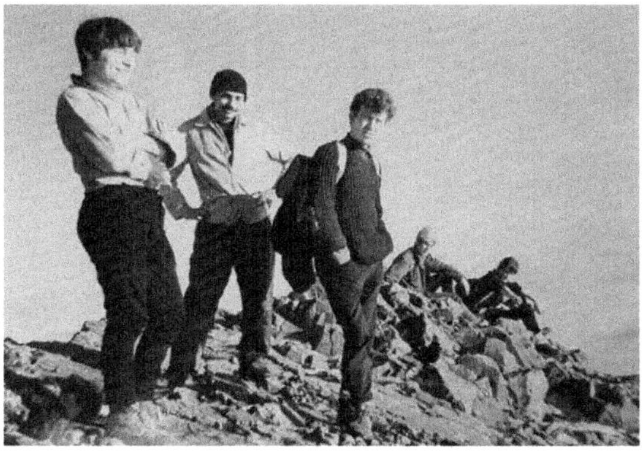
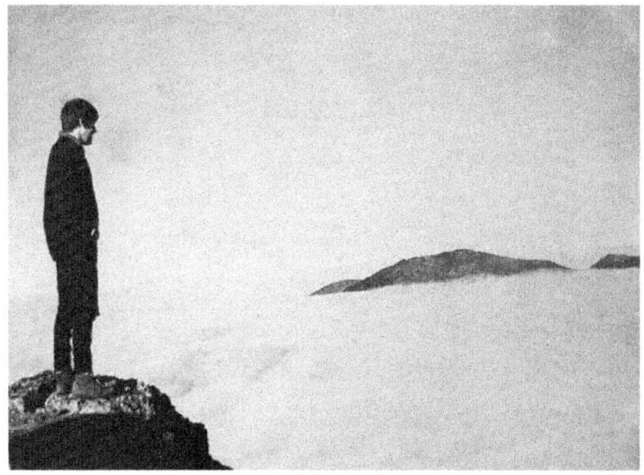

An exceptional day in winter 1967/68. Gary Rushton and Roger Bainbridge on Crib Goch looking towards Elidir Fawr. What these photos do not show is the very special halo/rainbow/shadow effect that was evident on the upper surface of the cloud. The photo below was taken about an hour later and shows the ridge between Snowdon and Lliwedd (Bwlch y Saethau) when the cloud formation was beginning to break up.

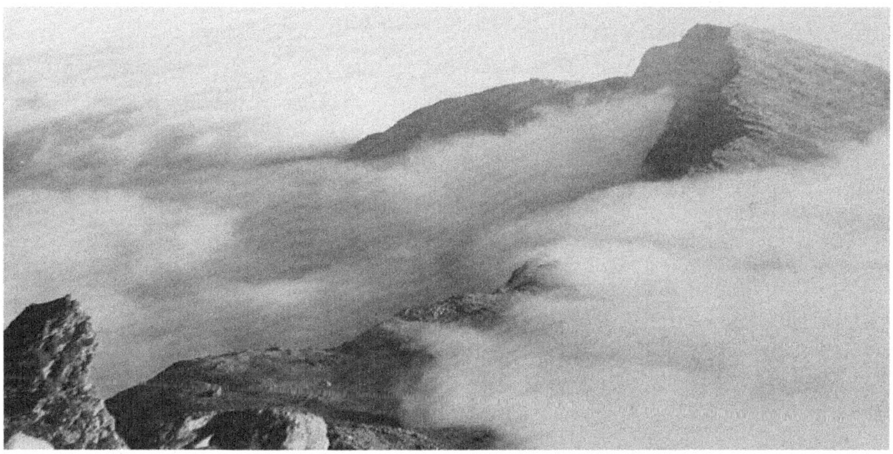

The following extract is taken from E G Rowland's publication 'Hill Walking in Snowdonia' and describes the effect as well as making reference to the link that this place has with King Arthur:

> The legend goes that King Arthur, having defeated his foes in the southern valley, drove them down towards Llyn Llydaw. Following them, the king was killed by a flight of arrows from the beaten foe. The misty monarch must have been as vital as a cat, judging by the number of places where he is reputed to have met a sticky end. A further tale says that a concourse of his knights lies dormant in a cave on the steep face of Lliwedd, waiting a trumpet call to renewed action.

While on Bwlch y Saethau you are not likely to meet King Arthur, but if you are very lucky you may observe a rare sight. In the late afternoon of a changeable day, when the sun is directly behind you and the vast basin below, that contains Llyn Llydaw, is filled with rolling mist curling near the tops of Y Lliwedd and Crib Goch, while rainbows come and go over the Glyders, there sometimes appears riding on the white cloud before you, a large shadow in human shape.

If you move from side to side the shadow does the same and if you raise your arms it follows suit. The special beauty of the spectacle is the oval halo that completely encloses the dark figure with full prismatic colours. This is the Brocken Spectre. It used to scare the peasants of the Alps as a manifestation of the devil, but over here a more kindly legend assures the observer of a front seat in heaven.

In 1967 the acquisition of driving licences, Austin A30's, minivans and Ford Anglia's ushered in a new era and most weekends saw us in the hut. I remember that we used to meet up in the snug at the Bell public house every Tuesday or Wednesday to discuss the next weekend's activities. Dates etched on the back of the Hut door told of our presence throughout that period but sadly, that record has now disappeared. During the autumn of 1967 there was an outbreak of Foot & Mouth disease. That didn't stop us travelling to the Old Boys Hut one weekend in the midst of the crisis, but Murray Watterson, who by then had taken over by the running of Plas, discovered us and we were promptly evicted on the Saturday afternoon. It was a couple of months before we were able to reclaim the Hut and resume our adventures there.

The following year Graham Dunn, Bainbridge and myself were back there most weekends. For several years we even took over the Hut for Christmas and New Year, the last one being in 1968/69. I know also that I was there for a three week stay in August 1969. That was probably the last time because autumn and winter 1969 was the lead up period to my finals and thereafter I went to work on a large construction project elsewhere in Wales. By that time, I had also met my future wife Judith, and her home in Porthmadog became the roof over my head when I was in the area.

Looking back on those years in the middle and late 1960s makes me feel warm and content. We had some cracking times in the Old Boys Hut and it was all the more satisfying because it seemed to belong to us; no one else wanted to use it. I conservatively estimate that I spent at least one hundred nights there, far more than I spent in Plas itself! Can anyone beat that?

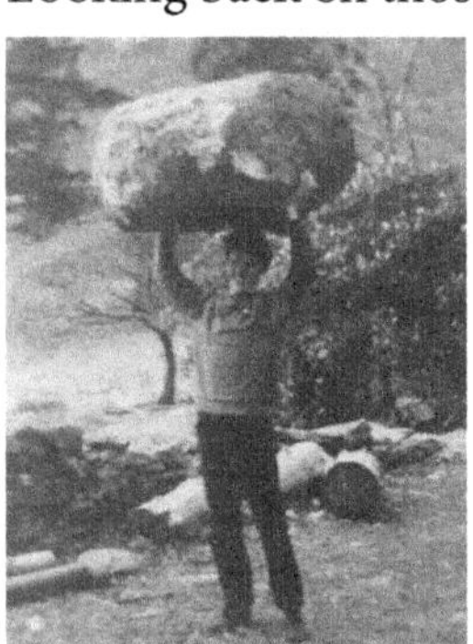

Left: Gary outside the Old Boys Hut in 1970, lifting one of the discarded polystyrene boulders, used in the Filming of 'Carry On Up the Khyber' which was released in 1968. Scenes on the North-West Frontier were filmed beneath the summit of Snowdon; the lower part of the Watkin Path was used as the Khyber Pass with garrison and border gate. In September 2005, a plaque was unveiled in Snowdonia to mark the spot of where the film was shot.

During this magical time there were significant changes happening at Plas. One change which I can fully approve of was the establishment of West Bromwich Mountaineering Club's Hut. During the early 1960s the building was an open-sided stone barn and I remember walking through it on the way to Eagle Rock. By 1966 front and rear walls had been added and it had become a fully functioning facility. My one and only stay there was in 1981 and it was very comfortable. My friend Graham Dunn joined their club and went to a number of their meets, (including The Globe public house in Reform Street) in order to obtain use of the hut for one weekend.

Another change which I suppose has to be considered beneficial was the supply of mains electricity to Plas Gwynant. I think this took place in 1964, about the time that George Simpkins tenure came to an end and Murray Watterson took over the day to day running of Plas. I list below, without comment, the other important changes that I observed:

i. Course type. Outward Bound style courses were replaced by learning experiences of shorter duration (now called Learning adventures)
ii. Building extension. Plas underwent a massive enlargement to accommodate increased numbers of youngsters and their teachers.
iii. Summer school camps. These were discontinued.

I suspect that all these changes were effectively complete by the early 1970s. I cannot be certain because, at that stage, other issues such as career, home building and children were occupying my energies and my time.

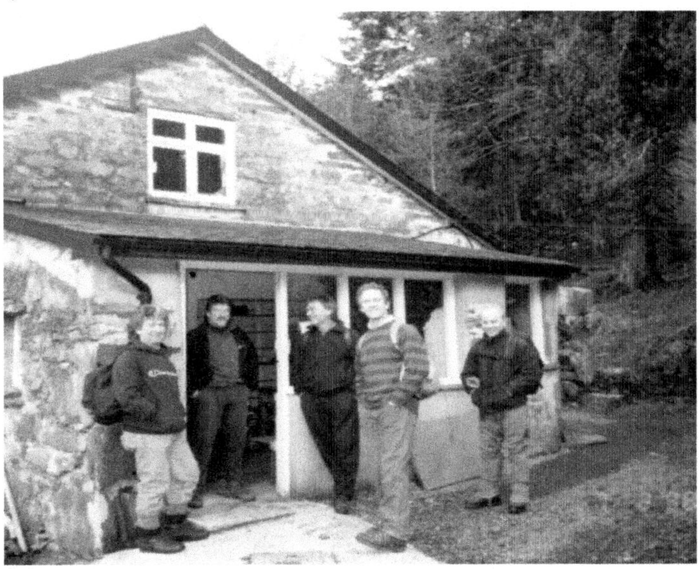

The 'Old Boys Hut' revisited February 1998 (Photo by Gary Rushton) L-R: Chris 'Rooster' Martin, (unknown in the doorway) Roger 'Bambi' Bainbridge, Roger 'Flash' Freeman and Ron Canty

Watterson retired sometime in the 1980s I believe but I am not sure who succeeded him. My occasional (unannounced) visits to the grounds of Plas throughout the 1980s and 90s made me think that as far as Sandwell youngsters were concerned, very little further change had taken place and the courses that went on within its walls continued to be of an educational type.

I did notice sometime in the 1980s that the Old Boys Hut had become the boot repository and the sign at the bottom of the drive had been replaced with something that referred to outdoor pursuits rather than adventure.

I also recall about this time being struck by the presence of two or three 15-seater people carriers! In my time at Plas there was a single long wheel base Land Rover which was used to pull the canoe trailer and to occasionally move loaded rucksacks and ropes around the countryside. Boys and girls were not chauffeured around but had to walk. I well remember the half-day slogs that I had to do from Plas to Tremadoc and Plas to Ogwen. Unbelievable as it may sound now, when our time came to do the Snowdon Horseshoe, we had first to tramp the four miles or so from Plas to Cwm Dyli Power Station and thence to Pen-y-Pass before starting the walk.

I continued to visit Snowdonia throughout the 1980s and 90s, repeating ascents, finding new scenic gems and hidden treasures and introducing my children to the joys of Wales and its weather. Using skills I had acquired at Plas and elsewhere, I even made a number of high level traverses across some of the lesser frequented mountain outliers in Snowdonia. These included the Cadair Idris range, the Arans, the Rhinogs and the Berwyns. Invariably these adventures would involve two or three nights out under canvas and a companion who was of similar questionable mentality as myself. The walks would not have been possible without the kindly assistance of my wife, who for the most part, took care of the necessary transport arrangements.

In 1995 my long-time friend (and most trustworthy and committed accomplice in nearly all of the adventures described so far) Roger Bainbridge, suggested that he and I and a few other firm friends should meet up once a year in Snowdonia. We began this arrangement by basing ourselves in the Dolwyddelan area and walking up Moel Siabod from the east side in heavy rain and mist. Since then we have held these reunions every year without fail in a variety of locations in Snowdonia, initially in January or February but more recently in September time.

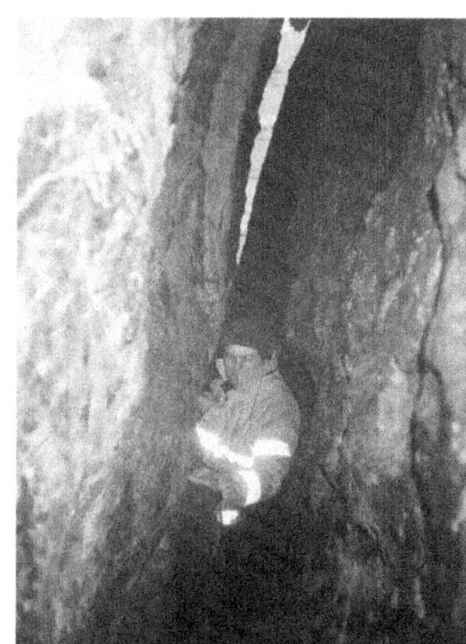

Above: Gary in Lockwords Chimney, 35 years after his original ascent

Not everyone can make it every year of course but Bainbridge, Chris Martin and I have not missed a single meet. And if that is not impressive enough, then bear in mind that Bainbridge, for the last twelve years or so, has had to travel from New Zealand on every occasion. Others who have come along from time to time include Trevor Clarke, Roy Simms, Derrick Lees and Brian

Hawthorn. The main reason I mention this event at all is that from 2011 to 2014 inclusive our accommodation was the Lodge that is located at the bottom of the drive at Plas Gwynant.

The Lodge was derelict when I first got to Plas in 1960 but it was upgraded and extended a few years later to accommodate Watterson and his family. Unfortunately, due to staff accommodation needs, the Lodge is now no longer available for hire.

In October 2010 I was wondering in the grounds of Plas Gwynant when I bumped into Jeff Handley, the current head of staff at the centre. I explained to him who I was and why I was sneaking about! He told me that I should go inside and speak to his admin person, Debbie Hughes. At the time Debbie was in the throes of organising a (delayed) 50-year celebration reunion event at Plas for spring 2011. Thanks to Debbie's splendid efforts this event duly took place and, by popular demand, similar events have been held every year since. These have given me and others the opportunity to make valued new friendships; for example, Wally Gough, Bill Hall, Frank Batchelor and Dan Jackson.

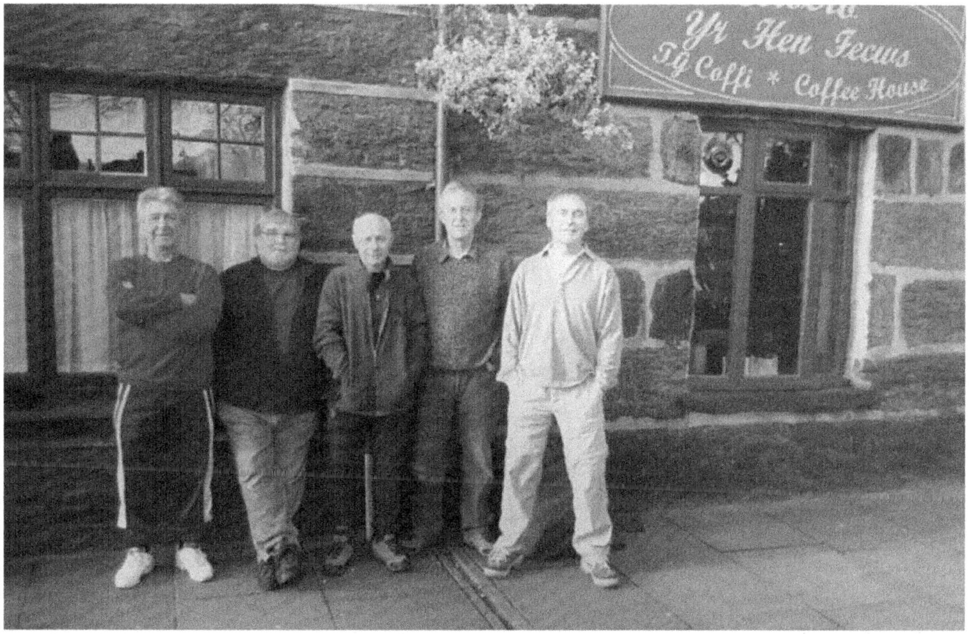

2005 in Porthmadog, outside the B&B Yr Hen Fecws
The gang: Chris Martin, Graham Dunn, Ron Canty, Gary Rushton and Roger Bainbridge

Next year (2018) it will be sixty years since Plas was acquired by West Bromwich and hopefully there will be another celebration weekend which I will certainly attend. I hope also that Plas will continue to provide inspiration to young people for another sixty years to come.

And so continues my long association with that little jewel that is Plas Gwynant and with what I regard as Britain's best National Park – Snowdonia. I count myself very fortunate indeed to have been educated in West Bromwich during the 1950s and 1960s and to have had the opportunity to experience both of these enterprises when they were in their infancy and were undoubtedly at their best and their brightest.

And it is satisfying to think that, through Sandra Meredith's herculean endeavours, not only have I been able to put on record my appreciation of that good fortune, but also to pay tribute to some of the marvellous friends who have been there with me throughout those years. How lucky I have been!

(Gary continues to attend the annual Plas Gwynant Reunions for those who came during the 1950's, 60's and 70's).

Chris Martin shares his memories of Plas Gwynant

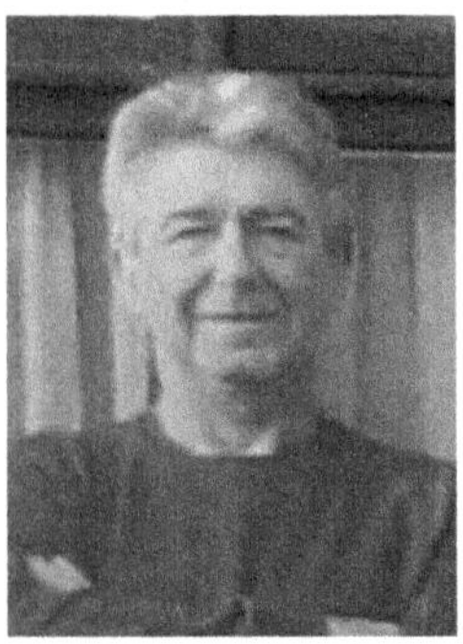

Strangely enough I never did an official course at Plas Gwynant, but did spend several occasions in the 'Old Boys Hut' together with Gary Rushton, his next door neighbour Ray Durden, Roger Freeman, Graham Dunn, Ian Bailey – like me, all from Yew Tree Estate – and Roger Bainbridge who lived in Great Barr. There may have been other 'Old Churchfieldians' from time to time, such as Roy Simms and Pete Reynolds.

Various parents took us to good hitching points, very popular in those days. In fact I never set foot in the house until the Sandwell Schools Reunions started! I remember the big cast-iron stove in the hut, which was very difficult to light and keep going – some nights were very cold. We did Snowdon, Horseshoe, various other peaks, climbing on Gladstone Slabs and also some abseiling.

I also remember swimming in the river some summer months. One weekend we hitched up on Friday and stayed in Willy's barn near Tryfan. We went to a nearby pub (I was around 16 years old), where I drank two pints of cider from the wood – I think a shilling a pint! I spent the rest of the weekend spraying 'diced carrots' on bales of hay, much to the disgust of the other occupants. Oh happy days!

More recently some of us have spent some great weekends in the Lodge – but cannot do that any longer it seems. Sixty year old friendships are still going strong thanks to Churchfields and Plas Gwynant. I really enjoyed my schooldays and was gutted when Churchfields was demolished. However, Plas is still going strong – and long may it do so.

(Chris continues to attend the annual Plas Gwynant Reunions for those who came during the 1950's, 60's and 70's).

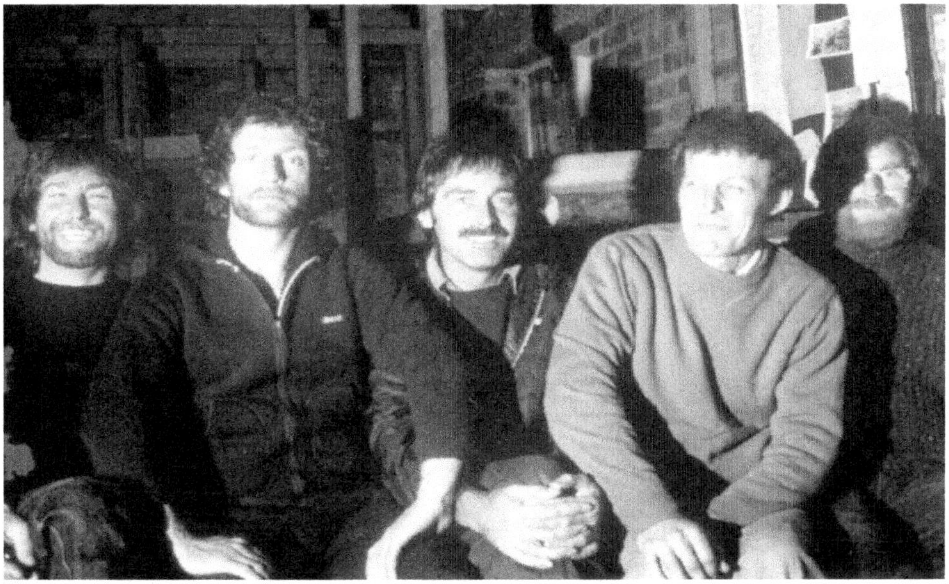

Chris Martin, Roger Freeman, Roger Bainbridge, Gary Rushton and Graham Dunn in the West Bromwich Mountaineering Hut, 1981

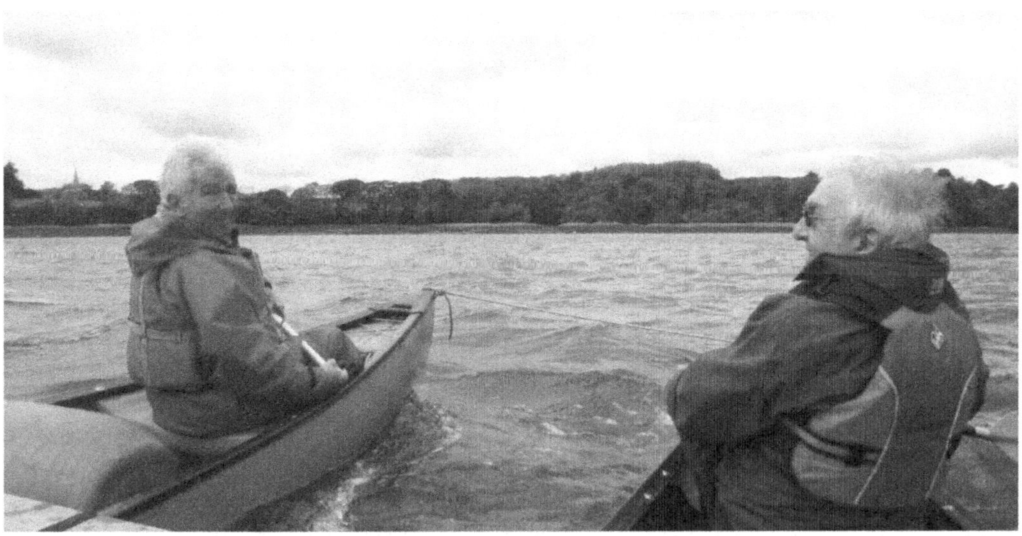

Chris Martin and Derrick Lees 2017 tackling the Swellies along the Menai Straits

Royston Simms shares his memories of Plas Gwynant

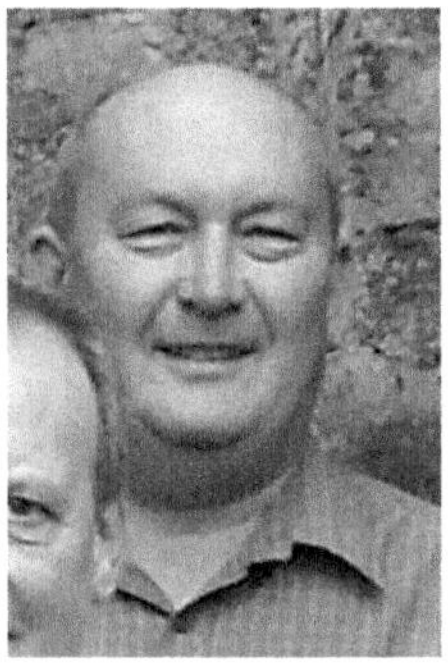

I was sitting in the library at Churchfields Comprehensive when in walked a school friend, Peter Johnson. I said "what have you done with your hair?" – it was a very short crew-cut. He explained that he had had it cut short for his visit to Plas Gwynant and that there was still some places left. "You should come", he said. "They do map reading, rock climbing, first aid, lightweight camping, walking, canoeing – and its only £5 for a month!" So I signed up for course number 26 in April 1962.

I was put into Ogwen Patrol with seven boys and never imagined in all my life that we would have such a fantastic time. Making new friends, learning how to look after yourself, share things and gaining a better understanding of a bigger world and an insight which would last you're a lifetime. In short, it actually changed my life.

There was no electricity in Plas Gwynant at this time; no phones, television or radio. Only self-entertainment at night, for instance Quizzes, games, reading, keeping a diary all by Tilley light. Olwyn the cook was magic! We had turns washing up, filling the Tilley lamps with oil, etc. Very early every morning we would run down to the river near the bridge, then all clothes off we jumped in the water! Out quickly due to the intense cold, quick rub down with the towel, got dressed and ran back for breakfast. This was the start of each day and it most certainly woke us up!

After four weeks our course came to an end, but not our thirst for more adventures, which resulted in many of us continuing our love of walking, climbing and camping for many, many years. Just over a year later I was asked to go on a second course and I was chosen to be a patrol leader, which gave me an unbelievable experience of being responsible for people rather than myself, which was a fantastic lesson in life. The positivity continued when my end of course reports were sent to me – included here.

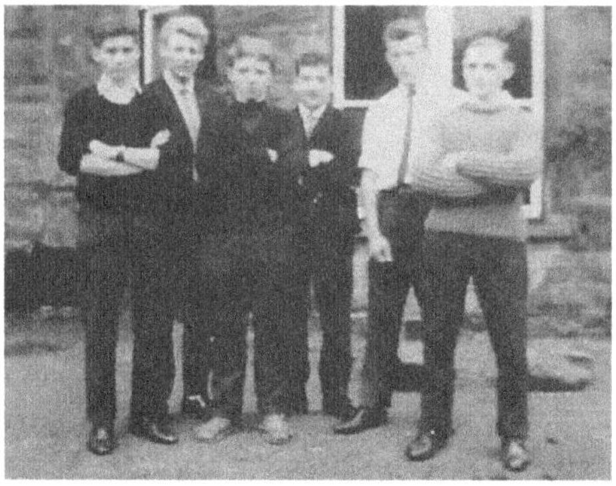

Above: 1963 – some of these lads had left school and were most likely to be an apprentice at a local firm.

West Bromwich Education Committee

Plas Gwynant Adventure School

REPORT

Name: Royston H. Simms

Age: 14.8

APRIL 1962

Royston is a quiet boy, fit, keen and very co-operative, who has maintained a high standard of enthusiasm, effort and achievement throughout the course. He was outstandingly interested in Map Reading and First Aid, asking intelligent questions and working on them in his own time. He stood up very well to the physical challenges of the course, camping, walking, and canoeing well and volunteering for extra Rock Climbing. He worked hard on routine duties and was outstandingly capable and reliable when trusted with unsupervised work in the canoe workshop. He spent an entire afternoon and evening of his free day completing a new canoe and showed a high standard of skill. He proved just as reliable at less congenial tasks and was altogether a most popular and reliable member of his group.

Name: R. Simms

Age: 16.1

AUG 1963

A tall, slim youth who has been to Plas Gwynant on an earlier course. Royston showed keenness and efficiency right from the start of the course and was made the Captain of his patrol. He led the patrol well and gained the good will and co-operation of all its members, setting them a good example of effort and enthusiasm and organising them well.

His personal work has been of a very high standard both around the school and at the various outdoor activities and he has volunteered for a great deal of extra work.

For the Long Day, the instructorless two day mountain expedition, his group was handicapped by a member with very painful feet but even so managed to complete a very creditable route of forty miles and eight thousand feet of climbing.

Royston was seriously considered for an Honours badge.

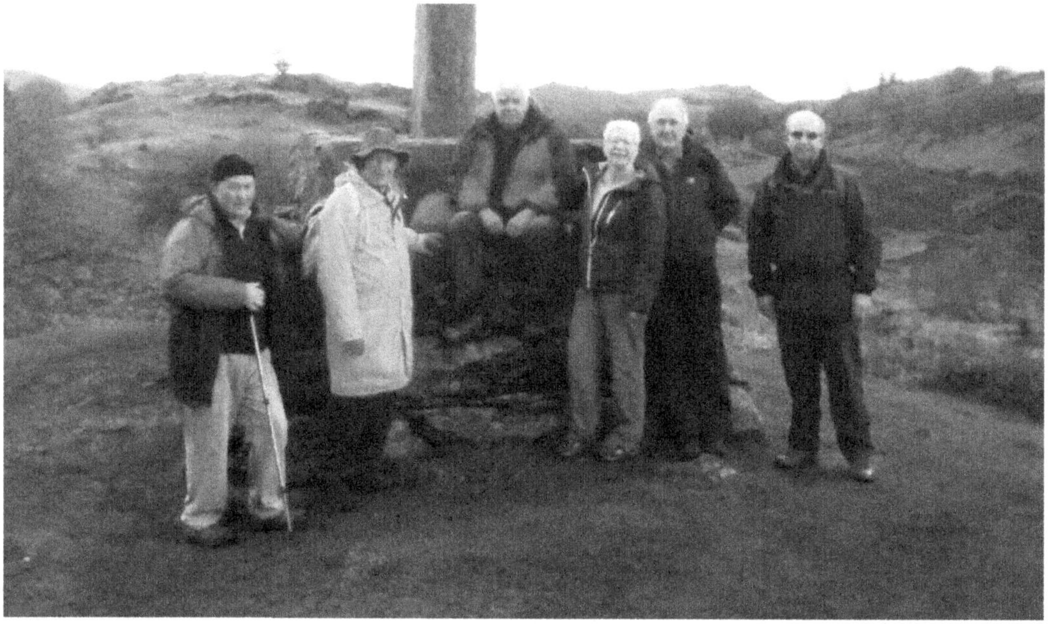

L-R: 2015 Reunion – Roy Simms, Gary Rushton, Bill Hall, Lynn Woodward, Derrick Lees and Roger Whitlock

(Roy continues to attend the annual Plas Gwynant Reunions for those who came during the 1950's, 60's and 70's).

Roger Bainbridge shares his memories of Plas Gwynant

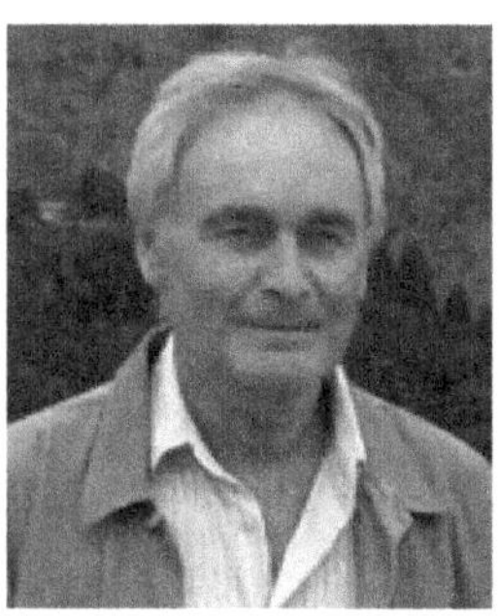

I attended Plas Gwynant three times in 1962, 1963 and 1964 at the same times that my friend Gary Rushton attended.
The first course in April 1962 was for one month and cost 5 pounds, which included all meals and was very good value. Boots were available to hire for 10 shillings (50p).

On arrival, via the bus from West Bromwich, we were greeted by the warden George Simpkin. Before we had to time to unload our gear he decided to take us on a run around the grounds, then down the road to the river Gwynant. He, with his faithful dog, 'Kipling', then ran across the cold river. We all stood on the bank looking. We had our city clothes on. Some of us tried to take off our shoes, but he insisted that we just run across as we were. The water was thigh deep! This was the start of quite a military style month at Plas. In fact I believe George had military experience and that's how he wanted to run things. Every morning we would get up a 7am, run 600 metres to the river and jump in naked. It was pretty cold. If you were a fast runner you could get there first and wet you hair and pretend you had been in. Sometimes you got thrown in by the others if you were spotted doing this.

We were placed in 3 patrols, Hebog, Tryfan, Ogwen, and were now in for a very competitive month. Every task we had seemed to have a points value and each patrol competed against the other. Even cleaning duties which were duly inspected by George and points out of 10 given. Sometimes someone in another patrol would sabotage your cleaning by throwing a bit of paper through a window after you had cleaned but before George had inspected. I was toilet cleaner. We had several other household tasks to do like lighting the Tilley lamps every evening as there was no mains electricity, in fact for all 3 courses I was on.

We did abseiling at Eagle rock on the premises which was enjoyable. We had canoeing on Llyn Gwynant and at Black Rock sands. Also did a first aid course. Rock climbing was a big part of the course. We had excellent instructors in Scottie Dwyer who was in his 60's but a great climber, also Terry Parker, Paul Hill and on later courses, Alan Hole and Dave Yates, (one of Britain's best climbers). We enjoyed the climbing and got up to climbing 'very severe', grades, which could be a bit scary but an adrenaline rush. We didn't have harnesses in those days, just tied the rope around our waist with a bowline knot. Also only belays over spikes of rocks. None of the modern day bolts and pegs. I used to visit Plas quite regularly and on one particular girls' course they let me take some of them rock climbing at Ogwen slabs. Something nowadays would not happen due to health and safety and insurance problems.
We had a thing called 'Potted Sports'. We were given tasks and had to overcome them, for example, using planks to cross a river. Also on some walks we had tasks to calculate the volume of water flowing under a bridge etc., all this again to gain points. Some of the walking expeditions were pretty tough. The 'Long Day', was hardest. Two days walking through the mountains with your patrol to find 'Clue Tins'. These tins were hidden and contained a clue word and when you found one it told you the co-ordinates of the next tin. We started very early in the morning and camped overnight sometimes in pouring rain and a full day again next day. You were not allowed to buy rations from shops, just take what food Plas supplied. Whichever patrol completed the course first and got all the tins 'won', the Long day. This was serious mountain climbing and was done at the end of the course. On one course two of the patrols gave up with mild hypothermia on the Long days. Not my patrol though, we completed all Long Days successfully!

On another walk in the Glyder mountain range some of the guys got exhausted and we had to carry the backpacks as well as our own. Good character building stuff. The second course in June 1963 was a month in length and also included some non-schoolboys. These were boys in employment and older than us schoolboys. Still no mains electricity, so still lighting the Tilley lamps. Again similar to the first course but we were bigger and fitter. We got to do even harder rock climbs which was great.

The third course in Jan1964 included kids from Marlborough College public school in Wiltshire, (very posh kids). This course was only for 2 weeks. We followed a truncated regime but still had the 'Long Day'. We had a ropes course that had to be completed by each patrol - again to get points. Part of this course required running along a plank and jumping through the air a fair distance to grab a rope to swing on. Unfortunately a Marlborough boy missed the rope and landed on his face from a height of about three metres and broke his jaw. The swelling was immense. That was the end of the course for him. Again no mains electricity on this course either. I think electricity finally arrived in late 1964. Ironic as just up the road was the UK's first hydro-electric power station. Apparently local villagers were against mains power for some time. (Following this course we were invited to attend Marlborough College for a week in the summer by the head teacher there).

Later in the sixties we were hooked on rock climbing and would visit Plas regularly and stay at the 'old boys hut'. This hut was actually a 'lean to', building on the old of the old barn used for storing equipment. Myself, Gary Rushton, Roger Freeman, Graham Dunn renovated the inside. There were 6 bunk beds and a fireplace which we put in in 1966 which smoked a lot!! There was a nearby water supply in an old lead pipe system opposite. The water was very brown if I remember.

Once George Simpkin left Plas for Tasmania I think Murray Watterson took over as warden. Courses got a lot easier, more leisurely. Not competitive at all. That's the way of the world now; can't take risks as afraid of legal consequences, which is a pity.
We certainly enjoyed the competitiveness and felt stronger and healthier following the courses. We felt we had achieved a life changing experience.

(Roger now lives in New Zealand)

Extract from the Churchfields school magazine 1964 by John Turton

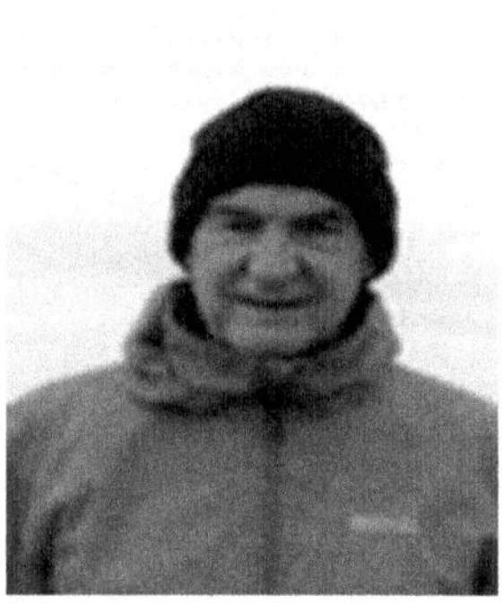

About twenty boys or girls attended a Norman course at Plas Gwynant Adventure School. They are divided into four patrols, each with its captain and own instructor. The morning begins with a dip in the nearby river and after breakfast each patrol carries out its duties on a rotary basis.

The first week is designed to teach the theory of mountain living and the use of ropes. This leads up to the first camp at Gladstone Rock during which the first rock climb takes place on Gladstone Slabs. In the second week, the ten-mile test takes place. This entails each patrol following a pre-determined route by map reading alone. In addition, course examinations now take place on the First Aid and map reading which has been taught for the first fortnight.

The third week begins with the Ogwen expedition during which three nights are spent in a barn and a climb is made on the Gribyn Rock. In addition to all this, an introduction is given into canoeing and abseiling; a ropes course is taken and initiative tests are held. Then came 'The Long Days' – the test in which everything that has been taught in the previous three weeks is used in practice.

After this stiff period, there is one day when the members of the course can choose which of the activities they have done in the past month they wish to do. Next day the goodbyes are said and the course disperses after an extremely worthwhile month.

William Hall (Bill) Shares his Memories of Plas Gwynant

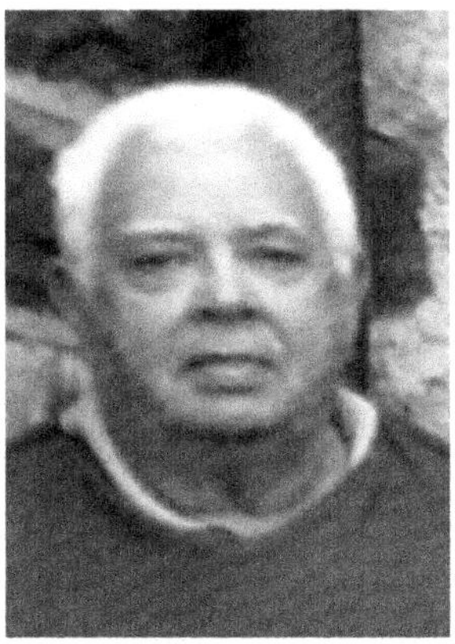

It was in 'A' Block at Churchfields when I first heard about Plas Gwynant. We were in registration when it was announced "who would like to go to an Adventure School for a month in North Wales?" The thought of a month with no maths, physics or chemistry was too good an opportunity to miss. I put my name down but was informed there were a limited number of places. Eventually I had a letter and met up with Mr Wright, who told me what was expected and that it was not a holiday.
The main points – boots, anorak, corduroy trousers, and, as I was in the Scouts, which was already a big part of my life, it seemed ideal, plus it was only £5 for a whole month!

The big day came and we met at Highfields, which in those days was the Education Department. Mr Wright was there and we were all told to behave on the coach and to go to the toilet before boarding, as we would only stop for a toilet break at Llangollen for 20 minutes. So off we set. I sat by 'Lettuce' Pete Leavesley, who was in the same set as me for some subjects. At Llangollen I remember buying a knife with the pound I found in my pocket.

I don't know what I expected to encounter in the deepest part of Snowdonia. On our eventual arrival at Plas we were met by this slightly framed gentleman with milk-bottle bases for lenses in NHS spectacle frames – this impression was extremely false. He turned out to be as sharp as a razor, strong as an ox and as fast as a mountain goat on the hills. He introduced us to the staff; Scottie Dwyer, a great father figure with the patience of a saint; Martin Endicote, who was a typical blonde athletic type, and Martin Riley, (short, slim and extremely fit and still don't know who he was).

After introductions we were allocated dorms – only the main building existed then. My dormitory was over the front door; names changed periodically and got swapped around, but Hebog, Tryfan and Snowdon were some. After this was the grand tour – drying room by the kitchen was really a draining room as there was no central heating, gas, coal or oil, only wood. A Tilley lamp used paraffin and was used early in the morning to give light before the diesel generator was started at 8.00am. At 6.30pm in the evening after food at Plas we would sit down to write our diary and write letters home. Diary would be checked each week and final assessment would be made at the end of the course.

We were taken down the drive to the equipment store and boot room for issues of petrol, fuel bottle, stove, tin opener, Blacks Good Companion tent, two sleeping bags: Blacks Icelandic, a Blacks Pal-O-Mine and a Blacks Ventile Anorak – far superior quality to my Millett! We then had tea whilst given our jobs for the first week. Mine was lamp lighting 6.30-7.00, so 9.00pm bed. This was an introduction that was to become one of the most memorable experiences a teenager could have.

We were woken up by a loud bang on the door at 7.00am. Grab vest shorts and plimsolls and run down the drive along road, over the wall and into the river under the bridge – return the same way! Breakfast, wash up and clean dining room. Then lecture about how to make a stretcher, erect tents, use the stove and cook dehydrated food, and anything else to make us safe and sound. To make sure that we were fully awake at this stage, we would have had a cold shower to wash the effluent off and sheep detritus from our emersion in the river. Every day at the centre our job would be one of the following:

Cleaning dining room, lamp lighting, toilets, showers, chopping wood, lighting the Aga at the crack of dawn so that we got a piece of glutinous porridge and a slice of bread and jam with a fair amount of tea that made builders tea look mild! On one occasion we were rabbiting after lights out when George Simpkins came up three times and told us to cut it out! The third time we were lined up outside in minus two degrees. No, we didn't need plimsolls to run to the gate which was 300 metres, then back again. This was a track not a road with typical Welsh stone surface; we hobbled to the gate as the stones were cold and sharp. We were glad to get back into our bunks before hypothermia set in and we did not chat again after lights out. (Poor bloke would be jailed nowadays. Yet we all felt okay about it as we were being a pain in the rear!)

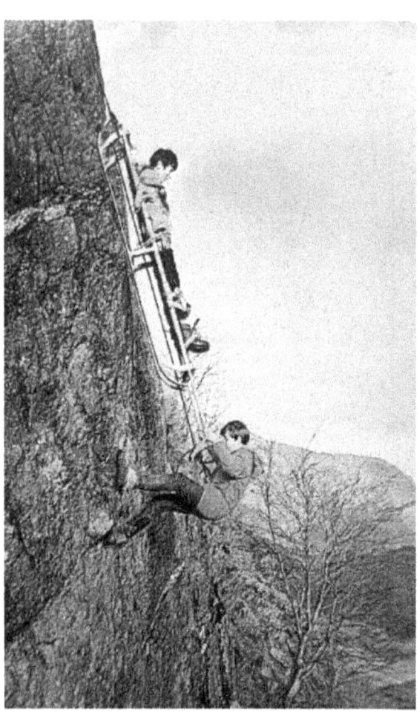

One phrase you never stopped hearing was the seven essentials – map, torch, compass, whistle, spare food, spare clothing and first aid kit.

Within the first week we were abseiling off Eagle Rock – a hundred foot cliff at the rear of the centre. At fourteen years old this was a new experience to all. If someone had told me I would jump off the practical block at school, the words I would have used would not be printable. But as ever, the enthusiasm and patience of Simpkins, you felt you could do anything. After we had all descended Eagle Rock it was time for our evening meal. Always a basic school dinner; mash, cabbage, meat and carrots followed by a slice of rice pudding!

On the second week we did stretcher lowering on Bryn Castle. This entailed jumping off a cliff tied to a stretcher, which was lowered by three points. This could end up with you spinning on the stretcher and if unfortunate, having your nose ground against the rock face, bringing tears to our eyes.

Week two was also highlighted by 'clue tins' when we were sent off in teams to find each tin at a certain map reference. The tin was usually in a hole in a wall, behind a tree or under a bush. This was three days under the shadow of Moel Siabod. On the second day we came across a fenced off area, which was consecrated. It transpired that in January 1952 in a blinding rainstorm, an Aer Lingus C47 Dakota aircraft crashed into Moel Siabod, a mountain 2,860ft high and burned out with the loss of all 20 passengers and a crew of three. Not all bodies were recovered and remains of wreckage and some of the dead were absorbed into the bog. It was strange why the plane was flying out of RAF Northolt to Dublin and plunged into the bog at the back of Plas in a place called Cwm Edno, which was a deviation from the standard flight path.

We also went down to Beddgelert and through the tunnel on the Aberglaslyn Pass. The railway track was a thing of the past and was just a sheep track. It was free entry to a copper mine - which was just a cave full of rubbish and let's not forget the tourist trap of the dog Gelert's grave for the more gullible English!

By this time we were getting more than capable of reading a map, lighting our petrol stoves – except on one occasion where a person, who shall remain nameless, decided to light the stove inside the tent because he was cold. He placed a little petrol on it to get vapour to rise. Vapour did rise because of the heat from the surrounding tent – which was on fire! This occurred during our solo. We were thrown out of the front door, given a map reference to cross mountains, get there and pitch tent, sleep, eat then return next day. We were all at different locations, though I did see the glow in the dark and heard the frantic yelling and someone doing a war-dance. I did feel sorry for him as we had one foot of snow that night – very cold and wet!

In week three our expedition took us up the Watkin Path where we camped near the slate works. This was to be a two-day expedition. On pitching the tent in the snow in darkness then melting snow for water, we put the vegetables in to swell. It was only when I went for fresh water for tea in the morning that I found a dead sheep in the water. This was the first night I tried to make chips with dehydrated potatoes – not a success!

The following morning we packed up and carried on to Bwlch y Saethau, down to Llyn Llydaw where we stripped off to underpants and boots around neck – Scottie Dwyer led the motley crew and encouraged us to wade through freezing water. We followed the hydro power pipeline down to the base of the Gwynant valley. We slept in a barn by the power house then the following day made our way back to Plas. (Pete never knew he drank dead sheep flavoured tea). We were then offered a chance to go canoeing and we all thought, great, no foot slog! It turned out worse as the canoes would have made an Inuit Eskimo or North American Indian say "White man stupid!" They were 14 foot long with canvas that was too heavy for a tall ship stretched over a wooden frame. They would have tested the cockleshell heroes! These vessels we had to carry to Llyn Dinas as we had no rights to go on Gwynant, so a fair lug on your shoulders. It took longer to get there and back than the actual canoeing. Martin Endicote came along in his Land Rover, asked "everything ok?" smiled and drove off.

By now we had got used to this way of life and thoughts of school and home did not exist – only the next challenge. However, on the second weekend we were allowed visitors. This was to enable anyone who wanted to jump ship if they wanted to. I think parents should have had a medal for driving the A5 with that much snow - this was in the days before motorway. Our next big expedition was up Gwynant Valley and over Glyders to Devils Kitchen from the Pen Y Gwryd hotel. This trip we were allowed to ditch tents as the load was too big for the distance. At this point we heard that the mountain rescue teams from Ogwen were out looking for a climber who got lost in a 'white-out'. This resulted in him losing his life and his body was found only 20 yards from the A5 in the snow at the base of Tryfan.

Dropping down into the Ogwen Valley we bedded down in a barn and the Land Rover arrived with extra rations. Next morning on the hike back, the weather was deemed too bad to cross the hills. This resulted in a route march to Capel Curig and then down to Pen Y Gwryd down a secondary road to Llyn Gwynant via the Gwynant Valley to Plas. Along this stage we had one member of the group exhausted and split his kit up for everyone else to carry. On reaching the gate to Plas, this was given back to him and nothing said. I have to say I was not enthusiastic about carrying someone else's burden as I think we were all cream-crackered! We had a day where we climbed Gladstone slabs, which I think most readers of this book will be familiar with. It has since become a point to where I always aim to have my sandwiches! Of course I am sure it is named after the famous Welshman who invented the Dr Gladstone bag.

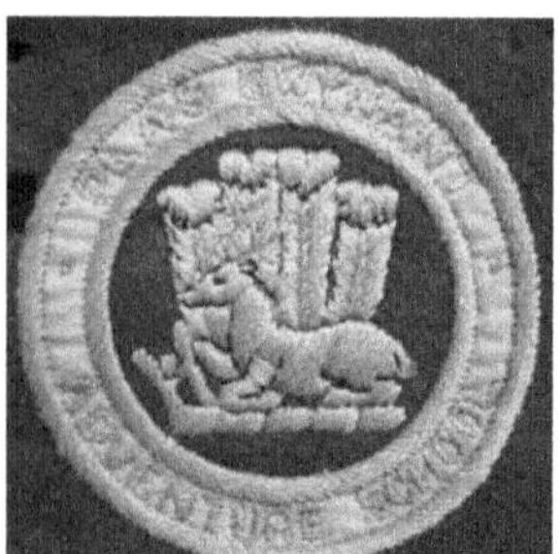

Our month was coming to an end; so much had happened it would take too long to write from the ungentlemanly peeing out of the window at night for fear of meeting the 'White Lady' ghost – and Martin Endicote at the front door calling his dog to come in from the rain. The throwing of a mortar bomb to each other that we found, saying if you drop it, you're dead! Simpkins jumping into a ditch shouting "are you stupid, it's live!" (And later the Army confirmed this!)

There were many more occurrences that happened on this memorable occasion and the fantastic staff. Climbing with Murray Watterson – who only three weeks before had admonished me in PE at Churchfields and was now Warden here at Plas. I had the privilege of working with him with a field trip course. Health & Safety – what's that? If it is burning and you touch it, you burn your fingers, if it looks dangerous, it probably is. For fourteen year-olds to wander around Snowdon unsupervised, people today would shudder. We had good instructors and you knew you had to listen. Acquiring your blue badge from Plas meant a lot. To get a different colour one you were lucky. I won't comment on grades of badges as we all knew who deserved red or green ones. All I would say is bring back self-reliance and team spirit where it matters! Thanks Mr Wright, Pat Tweedale, Murray Watterson and all those that have taught at Plas Gwynant and have gone to the great rock-face in the sky!

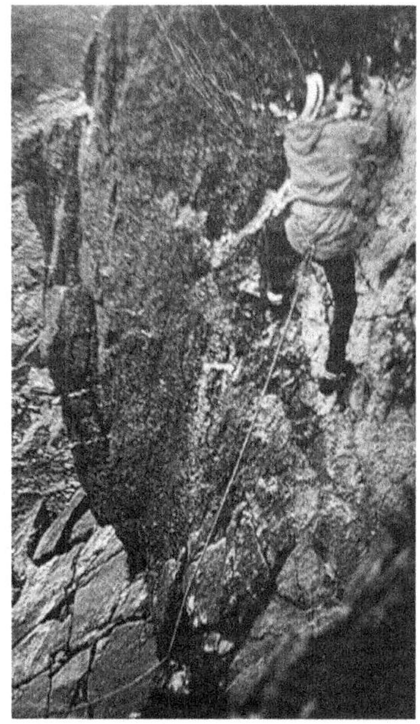

I was fortunate enough to go back in 1970 when Murray Watterson was boss. By now Plas had been swallowed up by Sandwell. However, I went with a group of pupils from George Salter School with a Mr Slee, who was head of Science; I was a field assistant. This was a field study trip for pupils learning about Biology, as well as studying flora and fauna with a smattering of Geology. On one occasion we returned after studying flora down by Llyn Dinas, to be met by John Roberts (Snowdonia National Park Warden) who wanted help, as a climber had fallen off the summit of Snowdon. I left the group who would now enjoy the warmth and comfort at Plas and proceeded in the snow up the Watkin Path, up past Bwlch y Saethau and traversing across to the left of the summit where we axed a platform in the snow for the casualty. Getting to the patient at the time is something I can only fantasise about now. Some forty minutes later the Plas y Brenin Team arrived from Capel Curig. We put him in a body bag and carefully traversed the face and got onto the Watkin and proceeded down. The RAF helicopter from Valley could not get down because of the wind and snow. It took about six hours to get him down but the distance was shorter than from the summit as he had fallen five hundred feet. Getting back to Plas at ten o'clock out of the snow and enjoying hot showers was a thing we did not know in the past; a leap forward into the twentieth century!

Everyone had the opportunity to go up to Gladstone Slab – brought back many memories. To be climbing with Murray and Daddy Dalrymple, the Scottish PE Master, who gave me so much grief in Rugby, and I think at some stage was head of Plas, seems strange. Murray Watterson to me always seemed a very fair guy and did his best to make sure the efficiency and ethos of Plas would continue into the future.

As I went around the centre, many memories came back but at the end of the week, I just think of how many urban pupils miss out on such a lot with such a short visit, with a structure that avoids any opportunity to show initiative.

Long live the Plas Gwynant spirit for those who still want to walk in the hills regardless of pills, artificial joints, creaking bodies – or wives!

As a footnote, one of the first people on the scene of the Aer Lingus disaster was climber and educationalist Ron Jones MBE, (a Brummie). It is thought that he walked on the wings to gain access. He, Trevor Jones and Tony Mason later set up the Ogwen Cottage Mountain School. Early in 1964 Ogwen Cottage was sold to Birmingham Education Authority where Ron remained as Chief Instructor for another five years. When Mrs Williams sold Ogwen Cottage, she gave instructions: 'In the case of an accident, fire a red flare in the car park to summon volunteers. When they arrive, pick the man with the cleanest boots to lead!'

I was very pleased to have spent a week doing mountain craft with Ron and in 1962 I was lucky enough to get sponsored to Ogwen Cottage to spend a week doing mountain craft, climbing, mountain rescue and map reading. Once again one had dedicated and highly professional mentors - Ron certainly being of them. However, I have been unable to confirm whether the story of the aircraft was correct but nothing about this man's determination and courage to help others would surprise me.

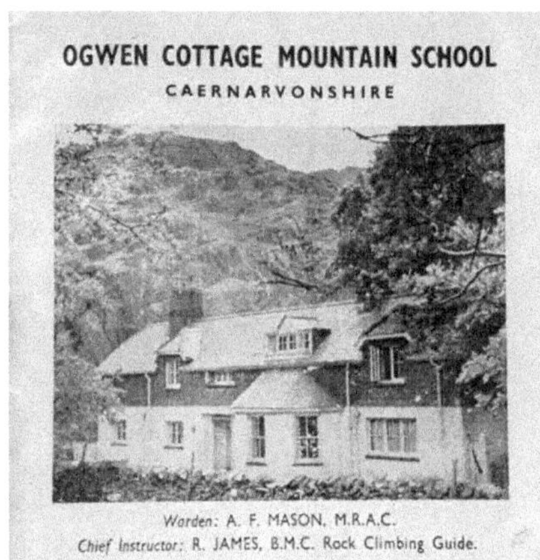

A 1950's brochure

Whilst I was at 'Oggie-Cot' I not only had a whole day as a one-to-one on the Carnedds on the trip down to Bethesda, but a day with Dave Yates, who was an instructor at Oggie-Cot at the time - we had a good time on Idwal Slabs. On leaving Ogwen Cottage Ron James and Ken Dwyer (son of Scottie), set up the Ogwen Valley Rescue Team. (Scottie of course was the very first mountain guide).

The King Charles pub at Capel Curig, later to become the Central Council of Physical Recreation at Plas y Brenin, was where students went for mountain leadership assessment - and for hot water and meals. Pen y Gwryd hotel was bought by Chris Briggs in 1947. This historical hostelry came to real fame in 1953 when members of the successful Everest expedition stayed there frequently. All signatories of the team are still featured on the ceiling. These, along with Ogwen Cottage are all mountain rescue posts.

(Bill continues to attend the annual Plas Gwynant Reunions for those who came during the 1950's, 60's and 70's).

~ IMAGES FROM THE EARLY YEARS ~

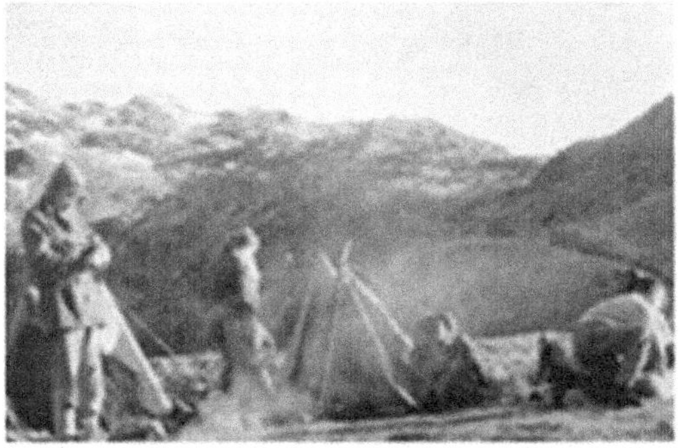
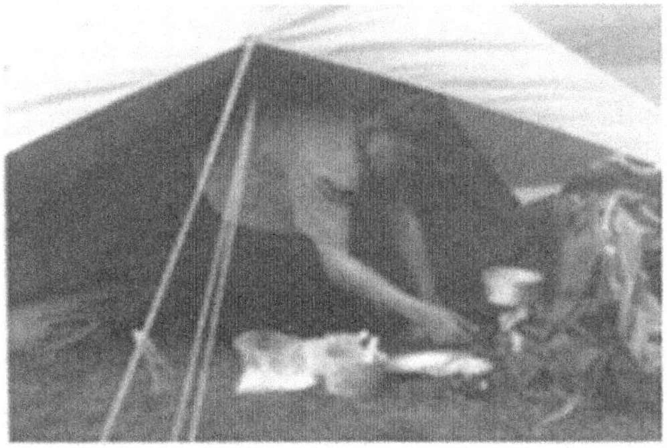
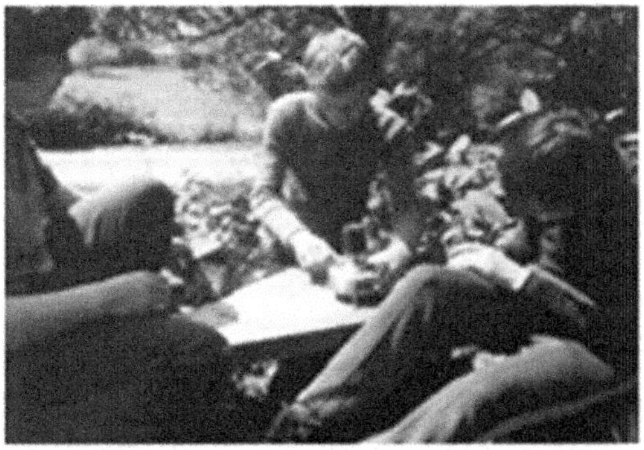
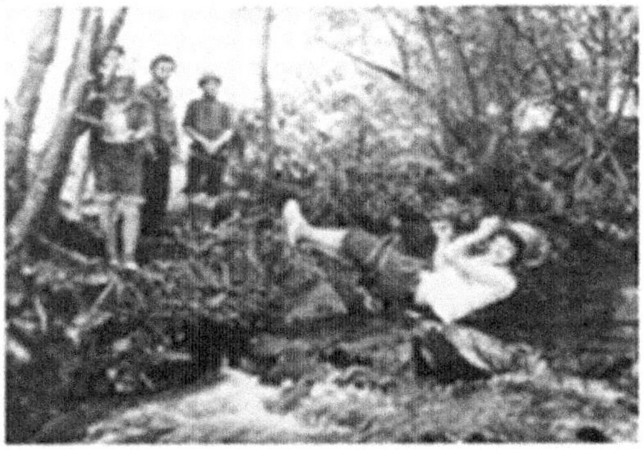
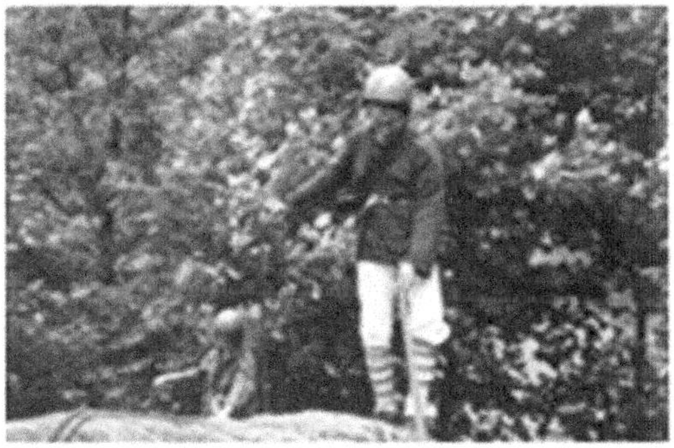
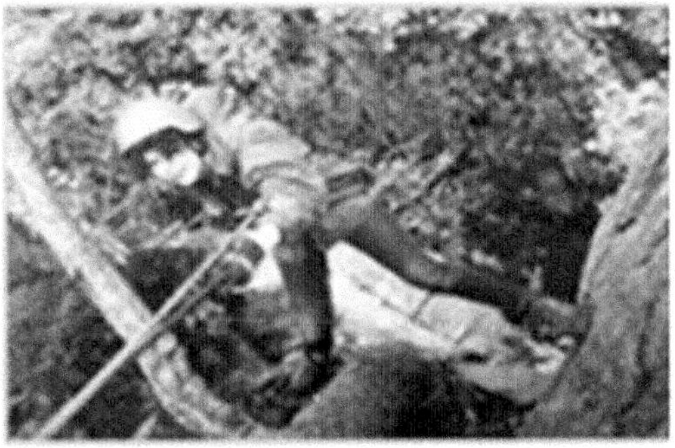
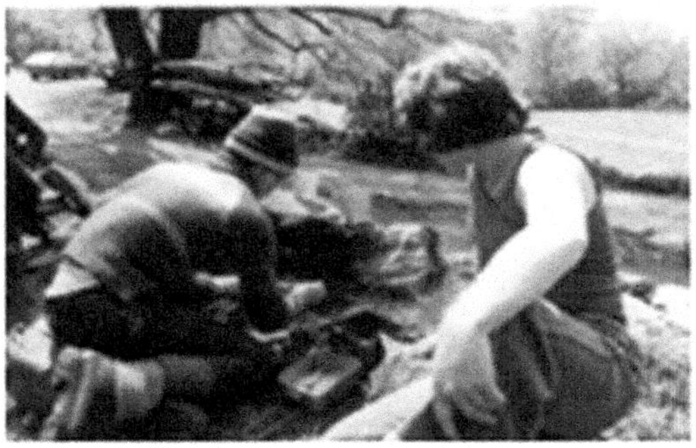
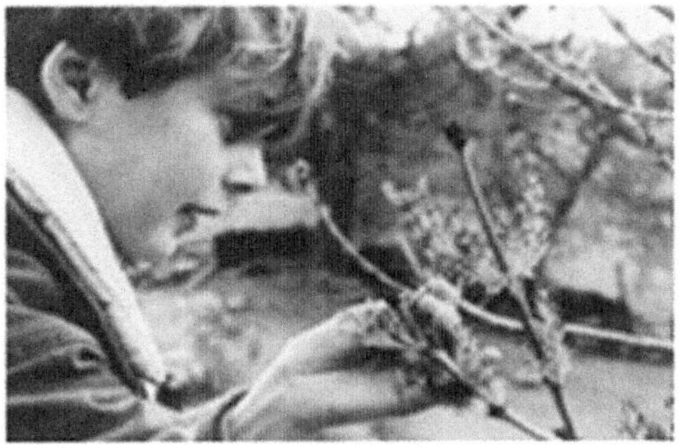

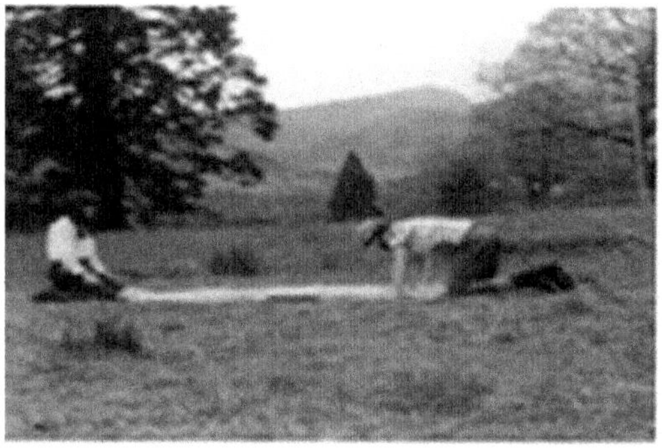
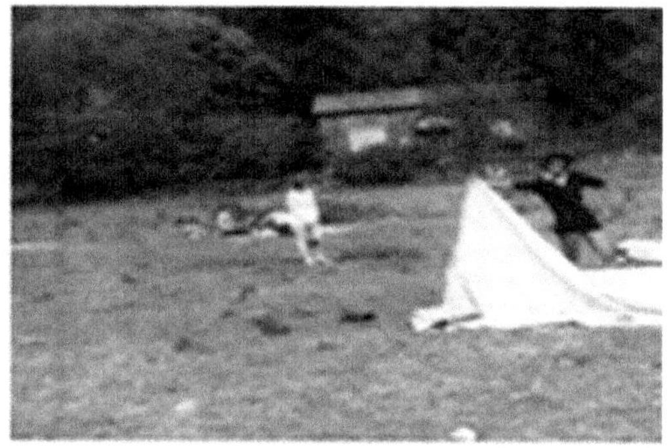
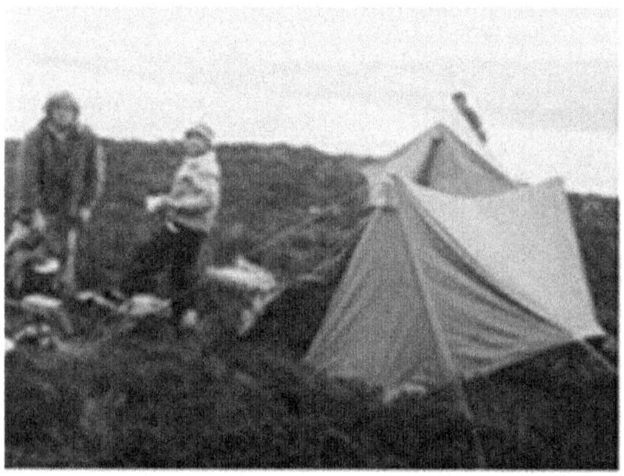
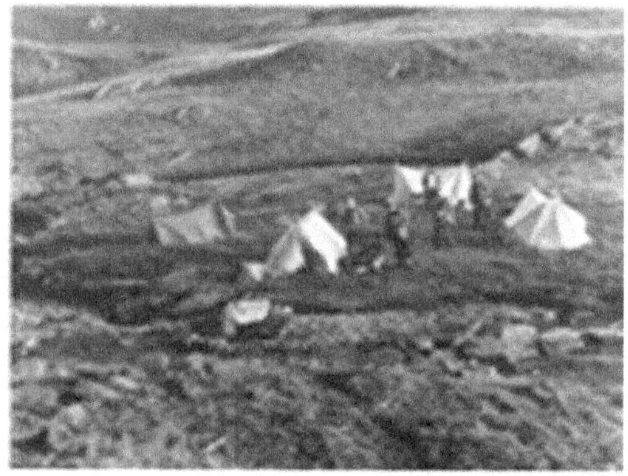
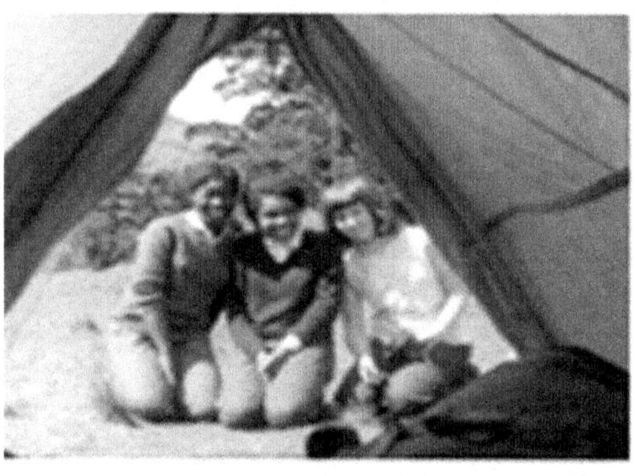
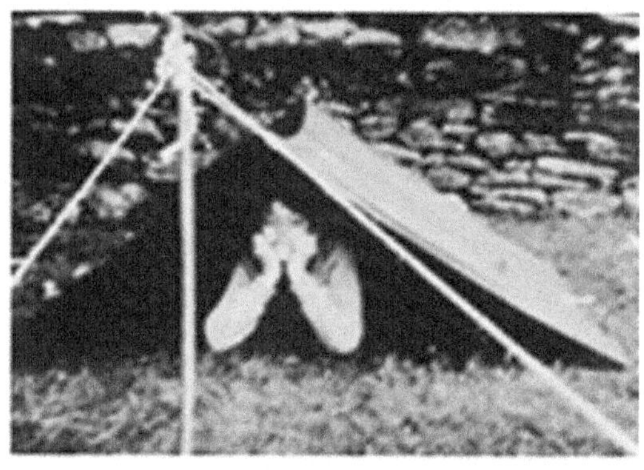
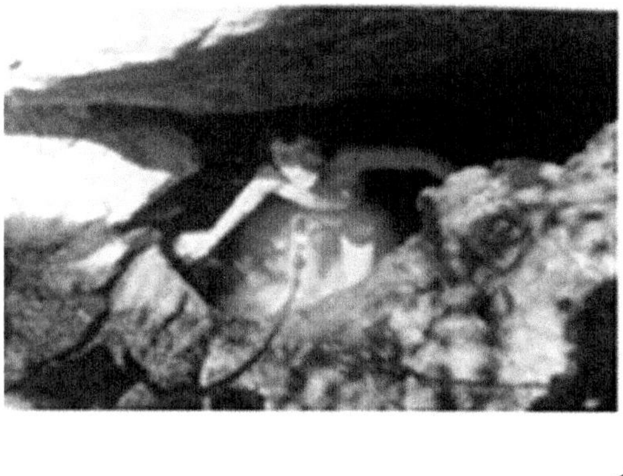
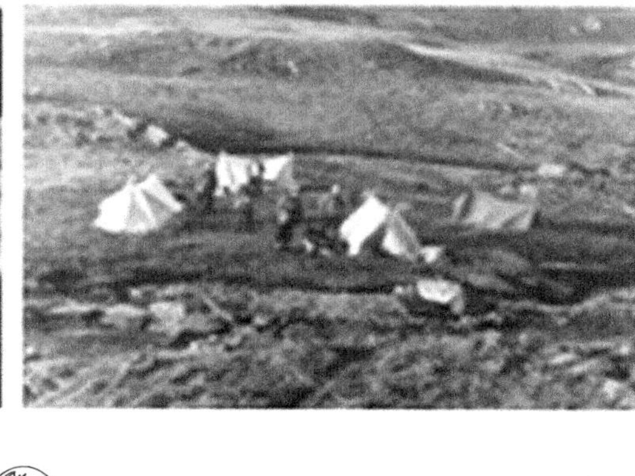

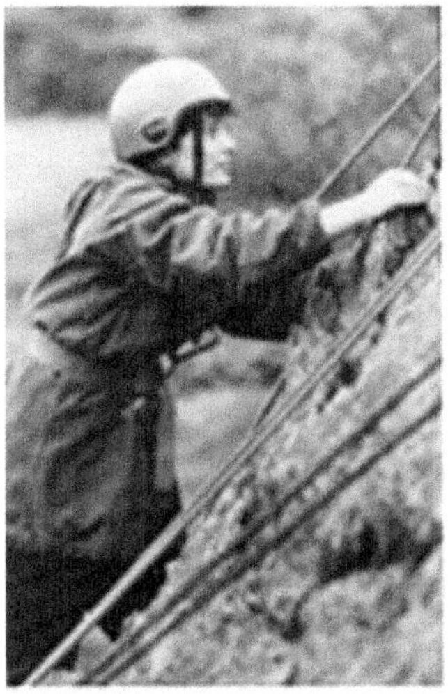

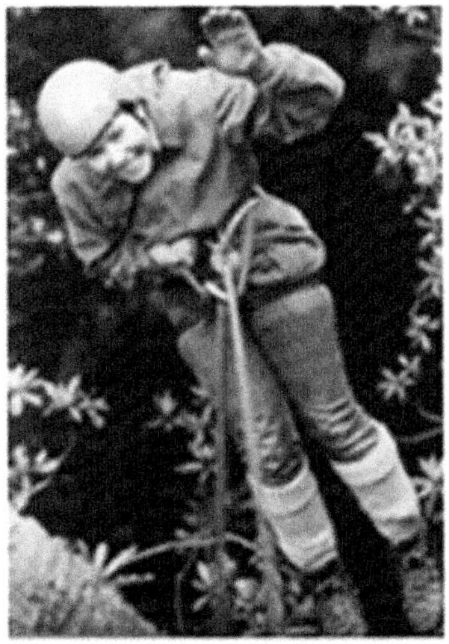

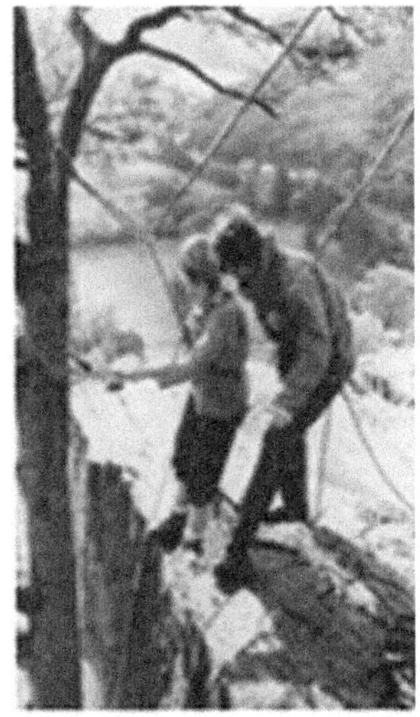

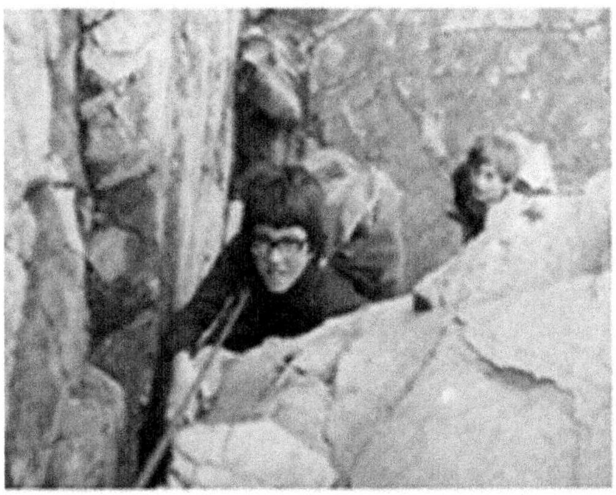

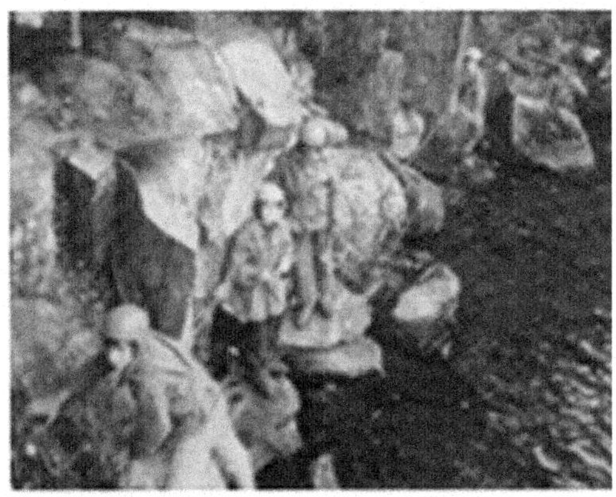

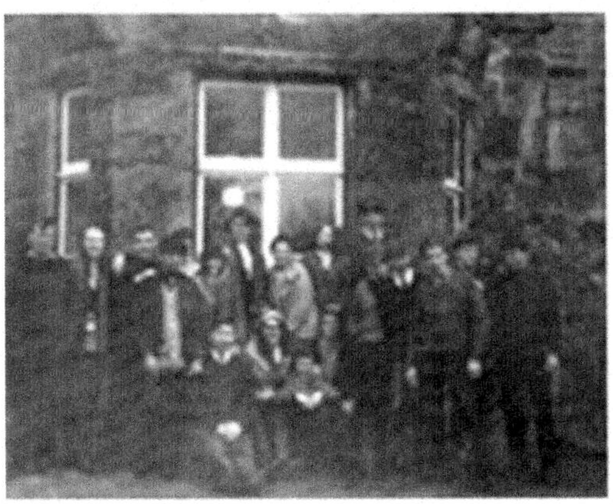

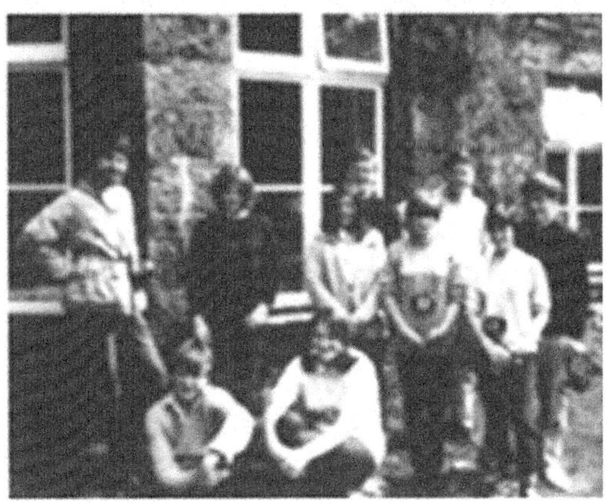

Two photographs from Peter Wharton, 1966 - with Murray Watterson Mary Bratt, Roger Morris, Mr Lance, Linda Ledbrook, Linda Broxton, Stephanie Bridges, Kevin Quiggan, Ramsay Smith, Richard Perry, Markham Kangure, Susan Ashbury, Olwyn Edwards, Garry Fenton, Peter Pugh, Mr Morris, Sheila Marti, Jen Hughes and Michael Wright

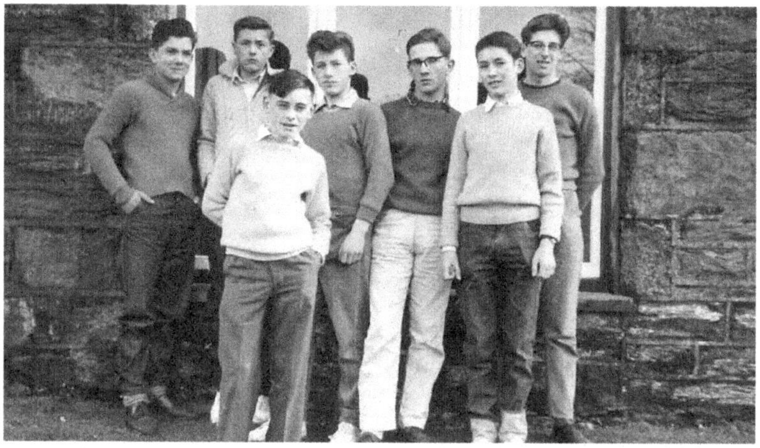

1962 with Rob Marshall (left)

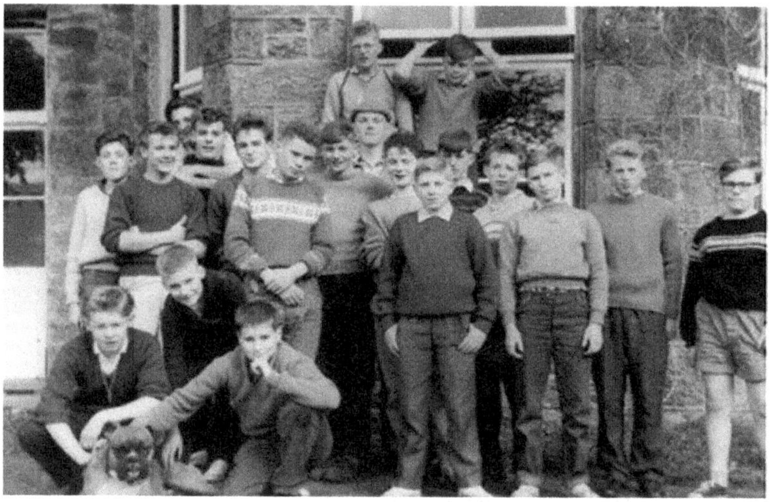

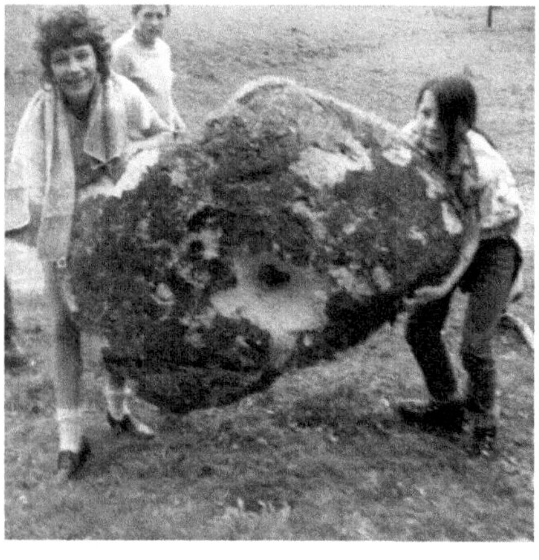

Fun with the polystyrene boulders left behind from filming 'Carry on Up the Khyber' in 1968

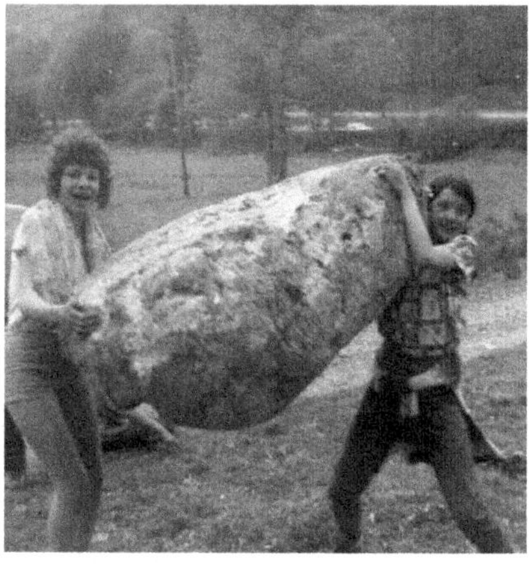

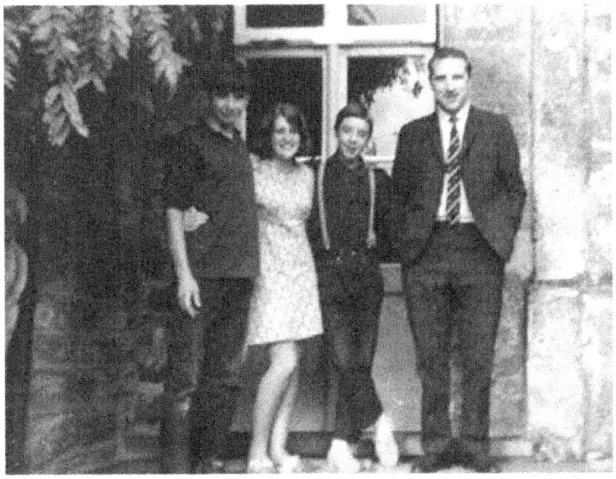

1968 Keith Jones, Elaine Silk, Francis Watson & John Allen (Churchfields Teacher)

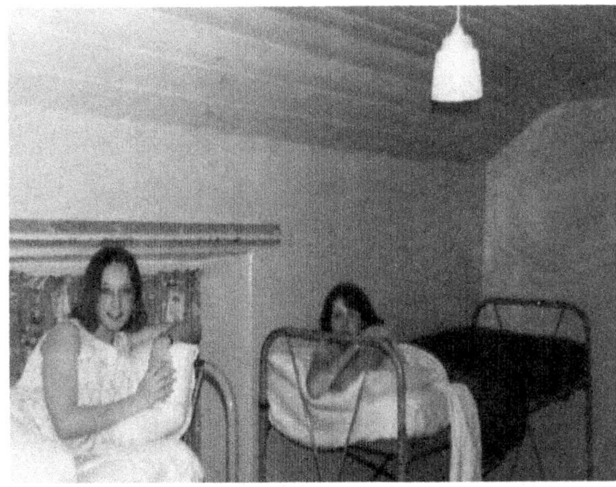

1968 Sandra Booty and Elaine Silk in the front bedroom above dining room

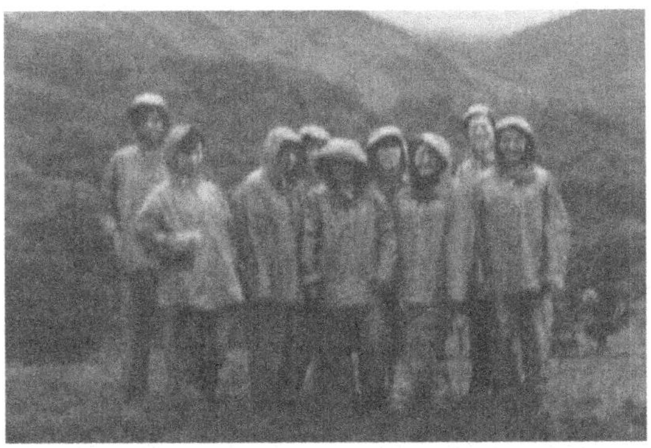

Judith Rogers (nee Charles) Lesley Cooper, Barbara Harrison, Rosion Charlton, Gillian Stokes, Marilyn Tonks (nee Smith), Wendy Wright, Jean Callaghan and Elaine Silk

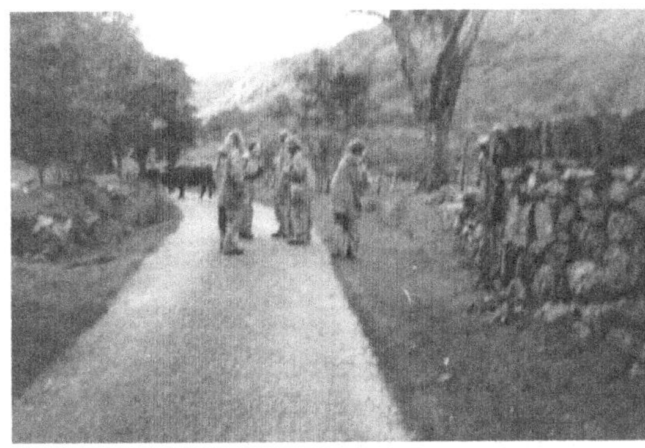

On the path to Llyn Dinas, encountering livestock obstructing our progress! Sandra Booty, Elaine Silk, Barbara Harrison, Judith Charles and Wendy Wright

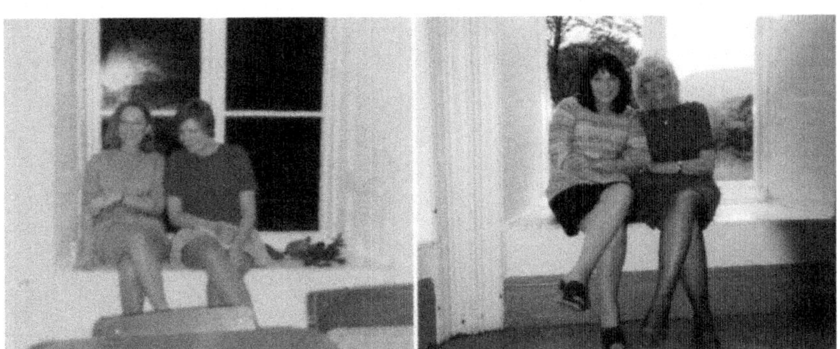

Judith Rogers (nee Charles) and Sandra Meredith (nee Booty) executing a 'before and after' photograph -1968 and then 45 years later at the Plas Gwynant Revisited weekend in 2013.

Sandra Meredith shares her memories of her visit to Plas Gwynant in 1968

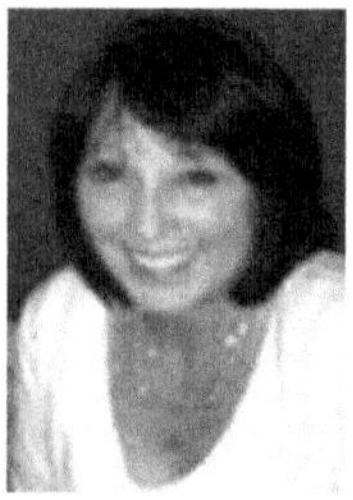

In 1968 Mr John Allen, geography teacher at Churchfields, supervised our class for a week long field trip to Plas Gwynant, which would form part of our exam marks.

In those days, many of us would either hate our teachers or love them – Mr Allen fell into the latter category!

I was happy to blow some cobwebs during our intense exam year, and maybe have some fun with my friends too. I remember the group of girls as I took a few photographs – their grainy remains are featured on the previous page. They are: Judith Rogers (nee Charles) Lesley Cooper, Barbara Ward (nee Harrison), Rosion Charlton, Gillian Stokes, Marilyn Tonks (nee Smith), Wendy Wright, Jean Callaghan and Elaine Silk. The boys I remember are Keith Jones, Francis Watson, Martin Bowman and Philip Cook (sadly can't remember others in the group).

We didn't sample the thrills of canoeing, abseiling, climbing or other appealing adventurous pursuits on our trip. For us it was mostly walking, taking notes, drawing sketches of a V-shaped and U-shaped valley, as well as studying the behaviour of the river as it meanders through the valley; cutting one side and depositing silt on the other! Mr Allen made everything interesting and I can almost hear him in my ear whenever I'm visiting Snowdonia. On one particular trek, my friend Barbara and I discretely mentioned to our intrepid leader that we needed to spend a penny. He obliged by advising us to go behind a huge rock while he kept the rest of the group engaged in his explanations about the source of the river and its journey. We returned to the group just as Mr Allen finished his talk with, "and Sandra and Barbara here are a perfect example of how a tributary is formed". Barb and I were mortified!

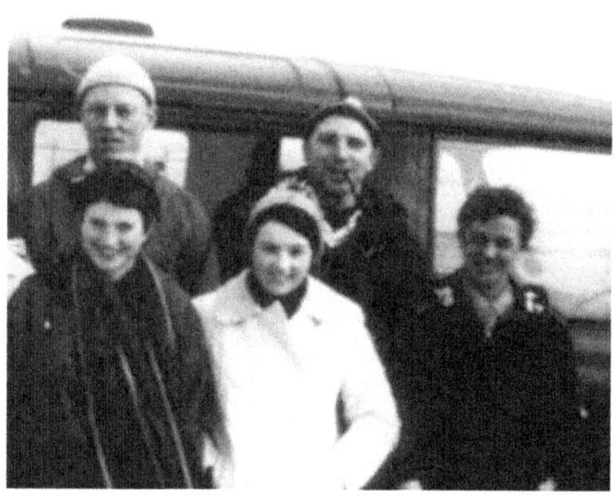

Mr Slack, Mr Allen and his late wife Muriel with two students

On another occasion our group stopped in Beddgelert where we enjoyed an ice cream whilst listening to Mr Allen relate the legend of Gelert the dog. A short walk south of the village, following the footpath along the banks of the Glaslyn leads to Beddgelert's most famous historical feature; 'Gelert's Grave'. The stone monument in the field is said to mark the resting place of the faithful hound of the medieval Welsh Prince Llewelyn the Great. The story, as written on the tombstone reads:

> *"In the 13th century Llewelyn, prince of North Wales, had a palace at Beddgelert. One day he went hunting without Gelert, 'The Faithful Hound', who was unaccountably absent. On Llewelyn's return the truant, stained and smeared with blood, joyfully sprang to meet his master. The prince alarmed hastened to find his son, and saw the infant's cot empty, the bedclothes and floor covered with blood. The frantic father plunged his sword into the hound's side, thinking it had killed his heir. The dog's dying yell was answered by a child's cry. Llewelyn searched and discovered his boy unharmed, but nearby lay the body of a mighty wolf which Gelert had slain. The prince filled with remorse is said never to have smiled again. He buried Gelert here".*
>
> Beddgelert Tourism

Many have since doubted the legend, but I still remember being transfixed on Mr Allen as he told the story to our group. This, and so many other teachings he imparted, managed to stay in my teenaged sieve-like brain, as well as a great fondness for this well-liked teacher.

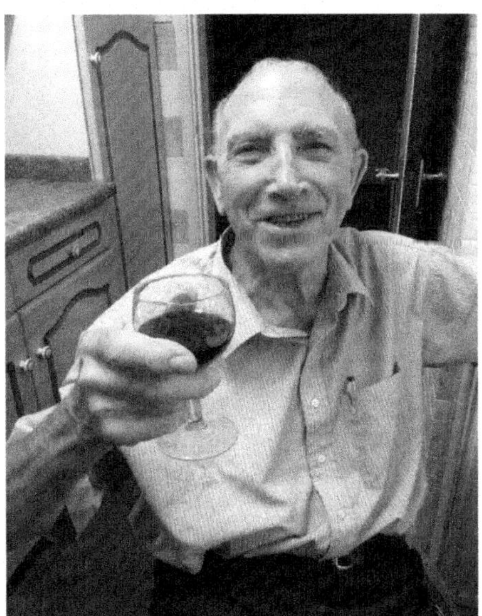

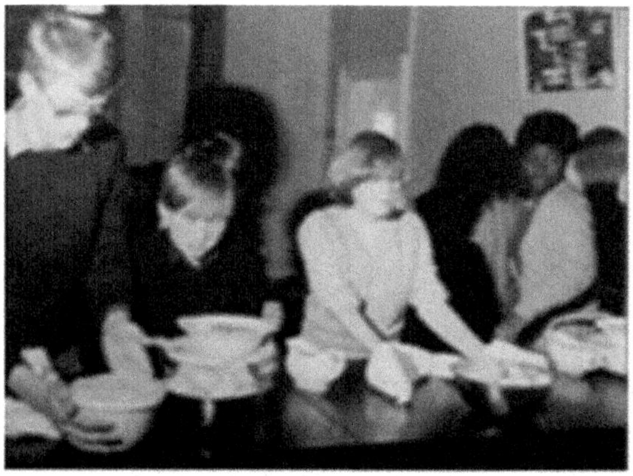

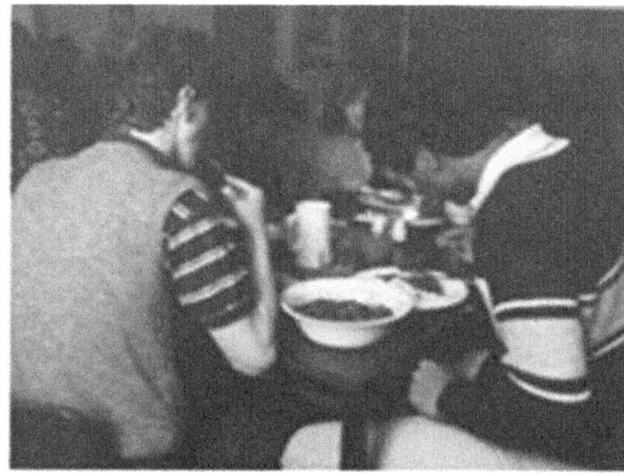

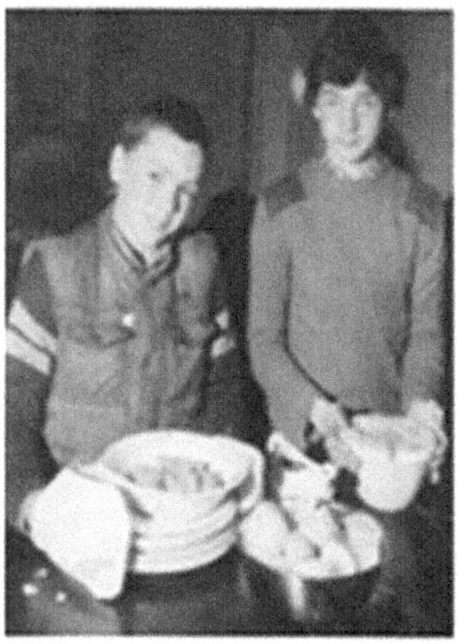

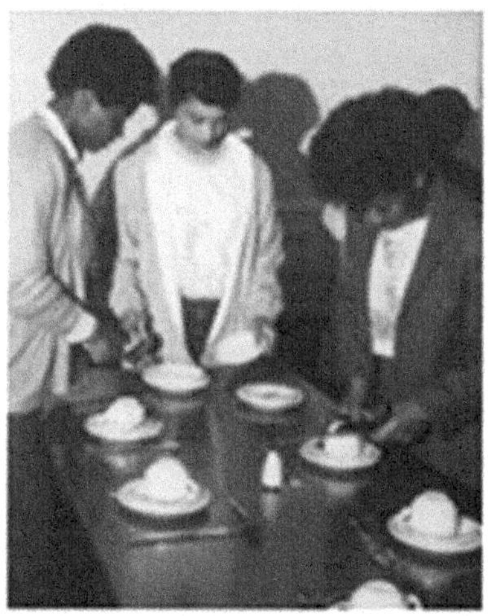

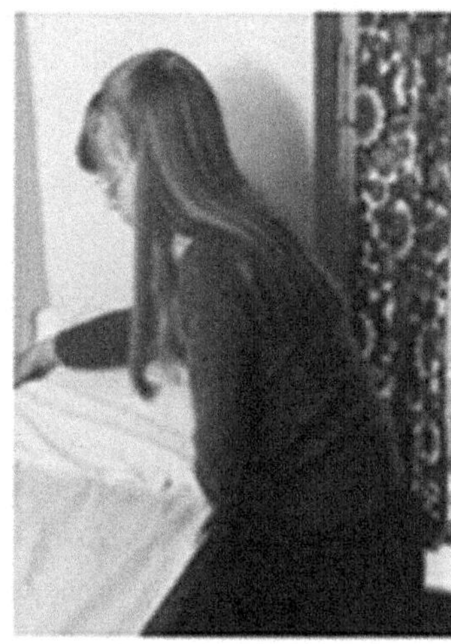

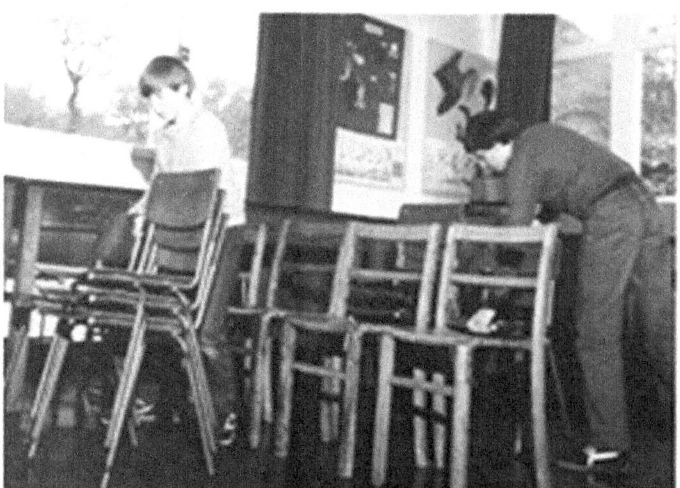

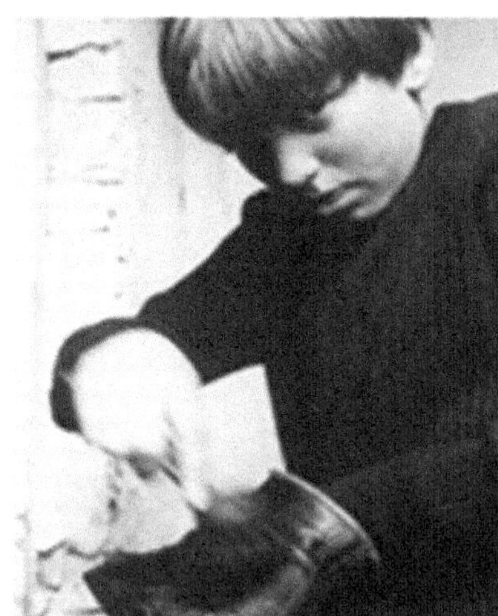

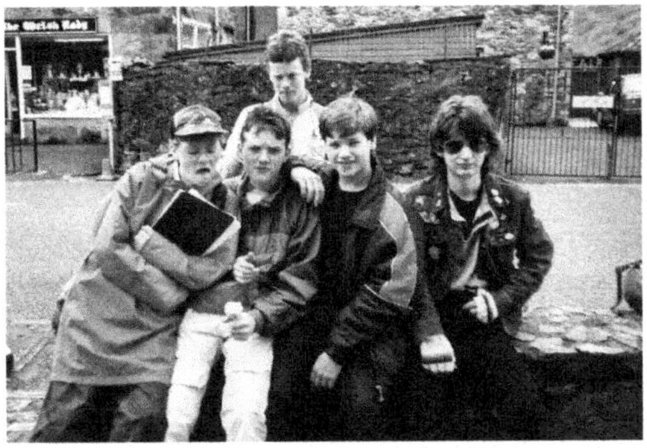

1987 Kerry Mander Scott Weldon Clarke Philip Ashley Hal and Brendon Blakesley

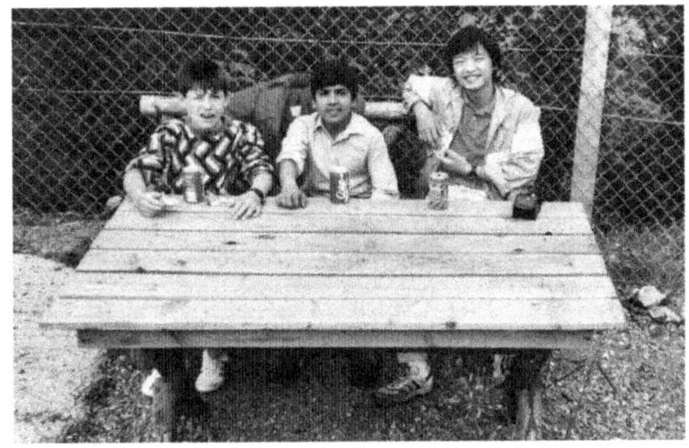

1987 Nicky Harris, Mohammed Fiaz and Trung Tre

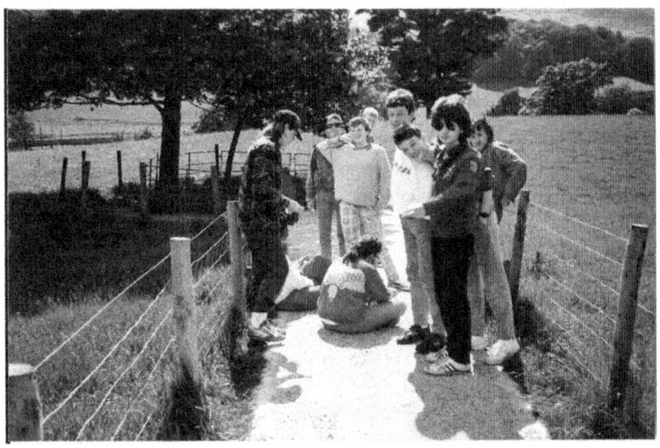

1987 Tracy Smith, Neil Woodfield, Clare Law, Kerry Mander, Grant Waldron, Clark Phillips, Scott Weldon, Brendon Blakesley and Michael Fisher

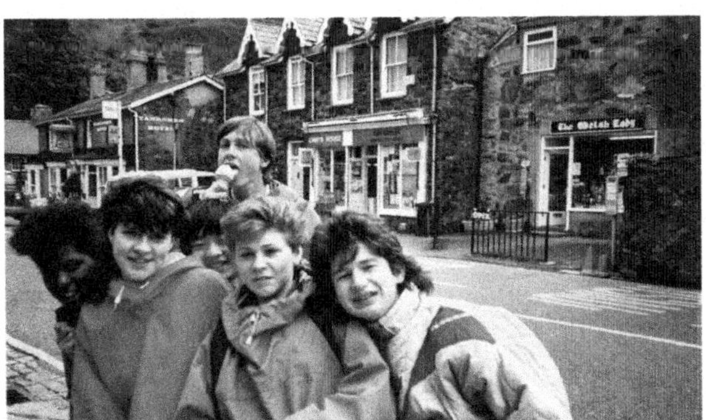

1987 Tracy-Delarosa Brae, Tracey Smith, Clare Law, Jason Hadley, Kerry Mander, Kerry Shrewsbury and Brendon Blakesley

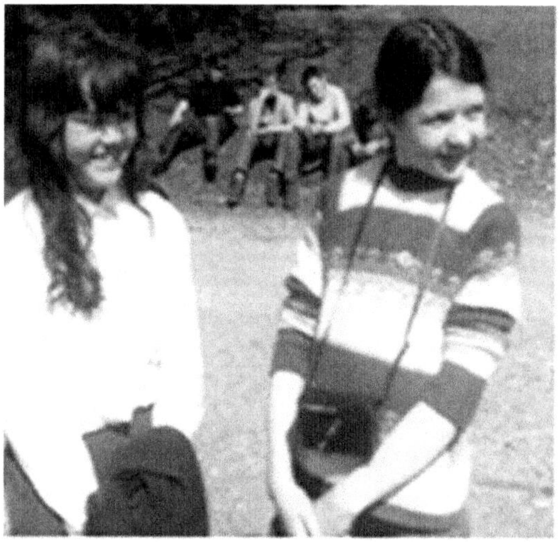

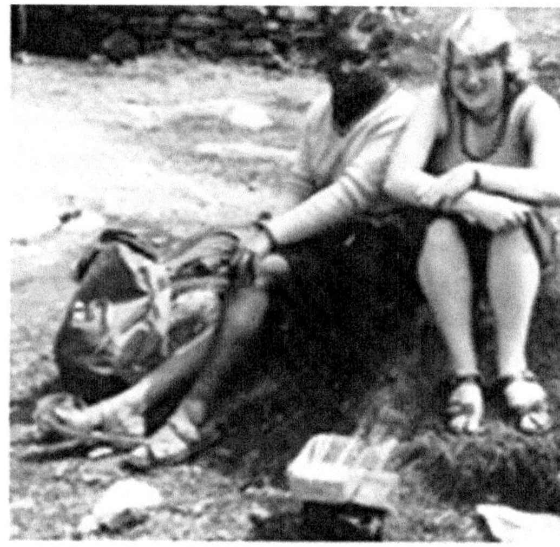

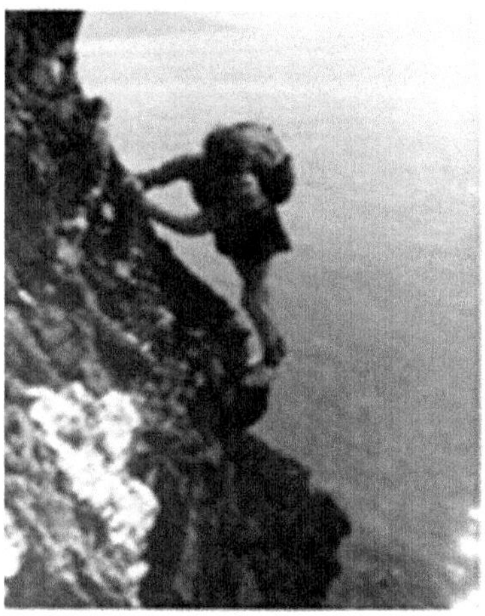

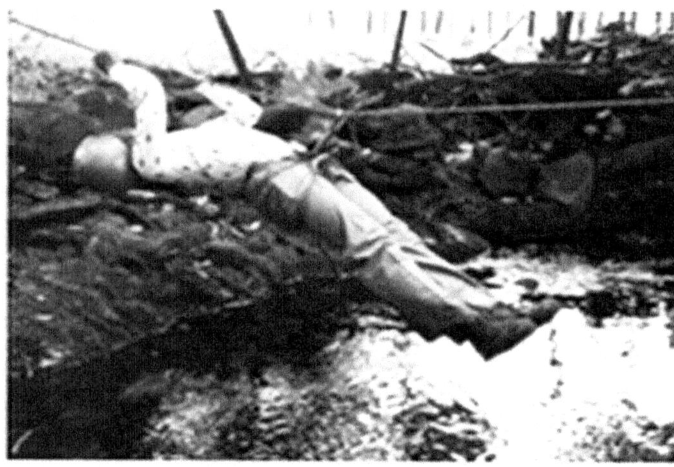

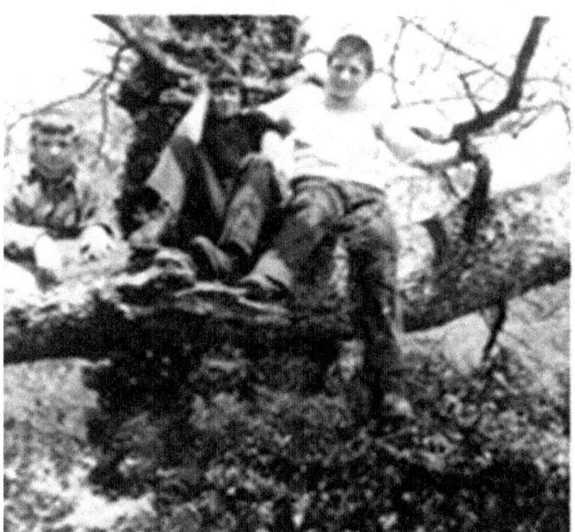

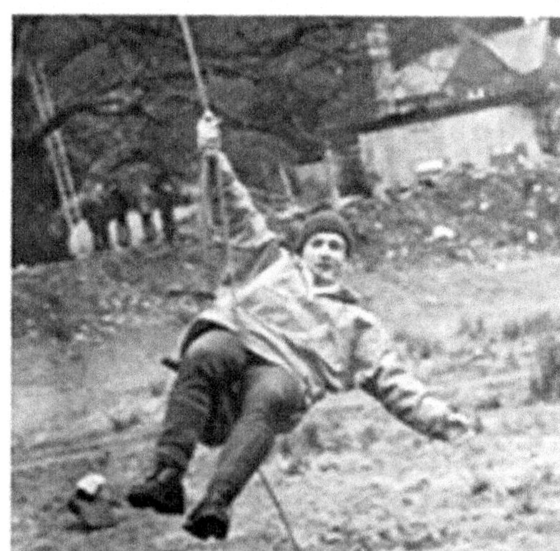

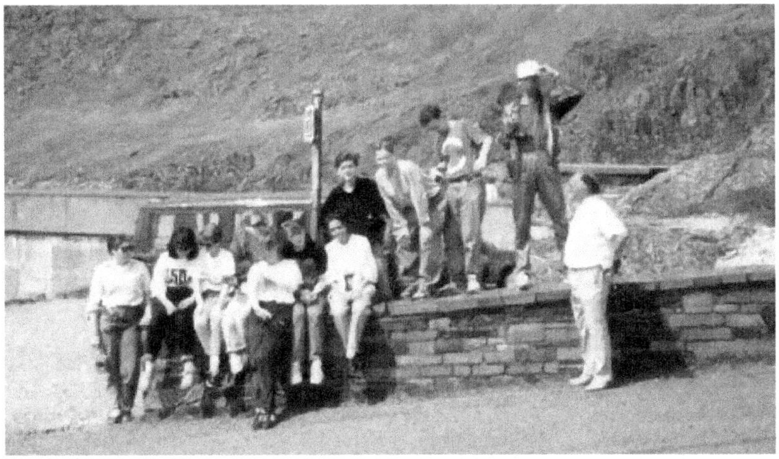

1987 - Samantha Kay, Heather Blakesley, Michelle Creswell, Alison Stokes, Catherine Richards, Helena Best, Davinder Kaur, Kevin Baker, Stuart Bailey, Stuart Upton, Paul Sidhu and Norman Whittington

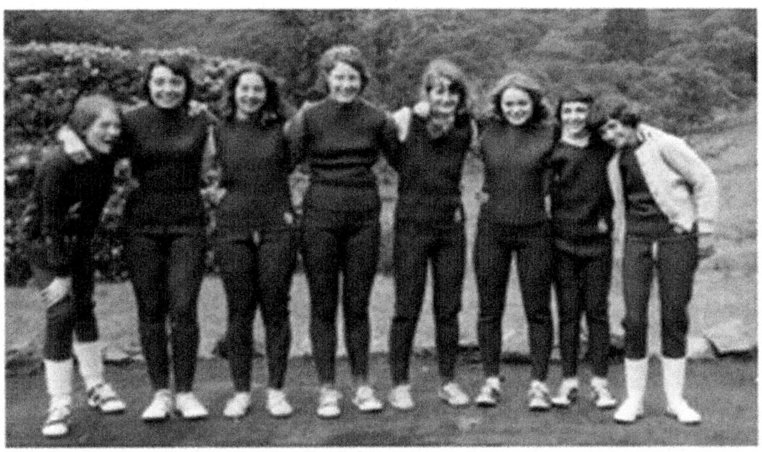

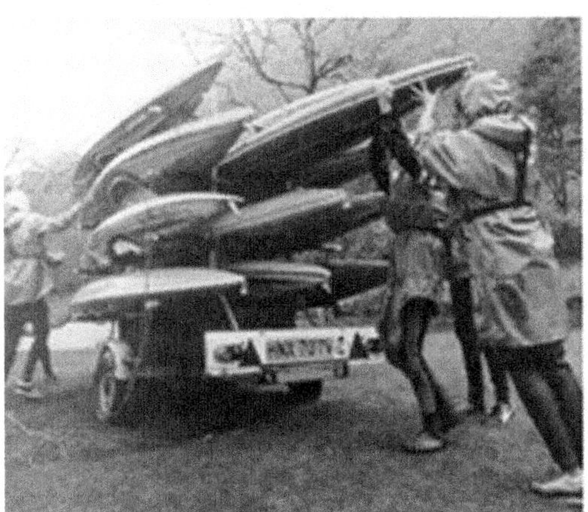

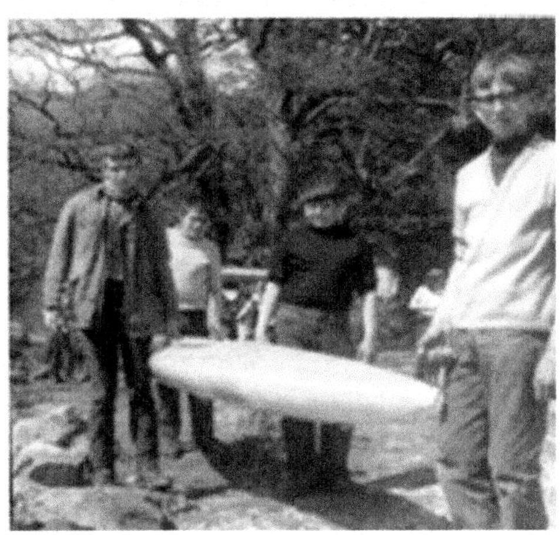

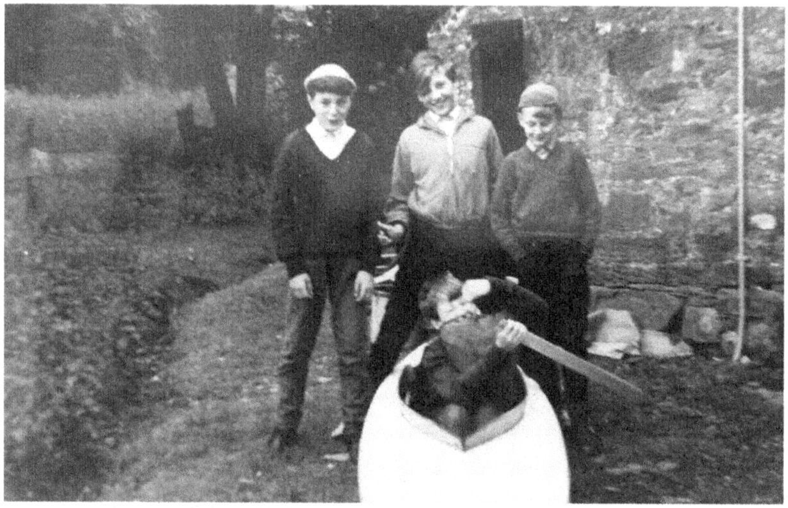

Above: 1963- Michael Reynolds, Micky Banner and Jimmy Willis and Nick Bowbanks in canoe

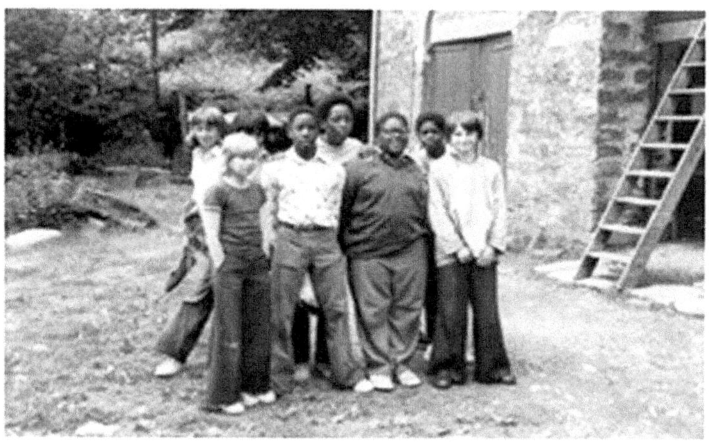

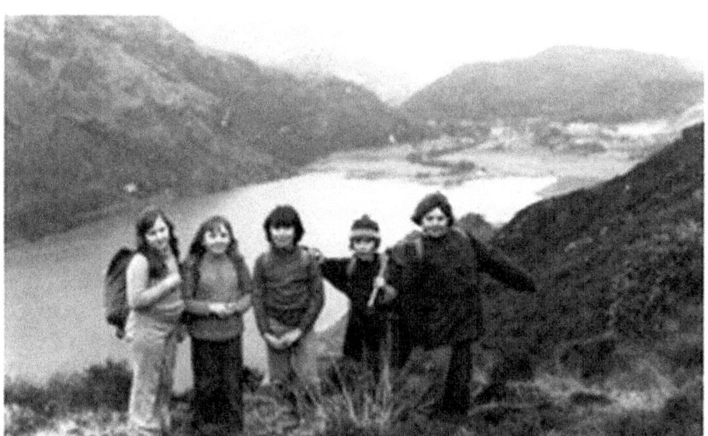

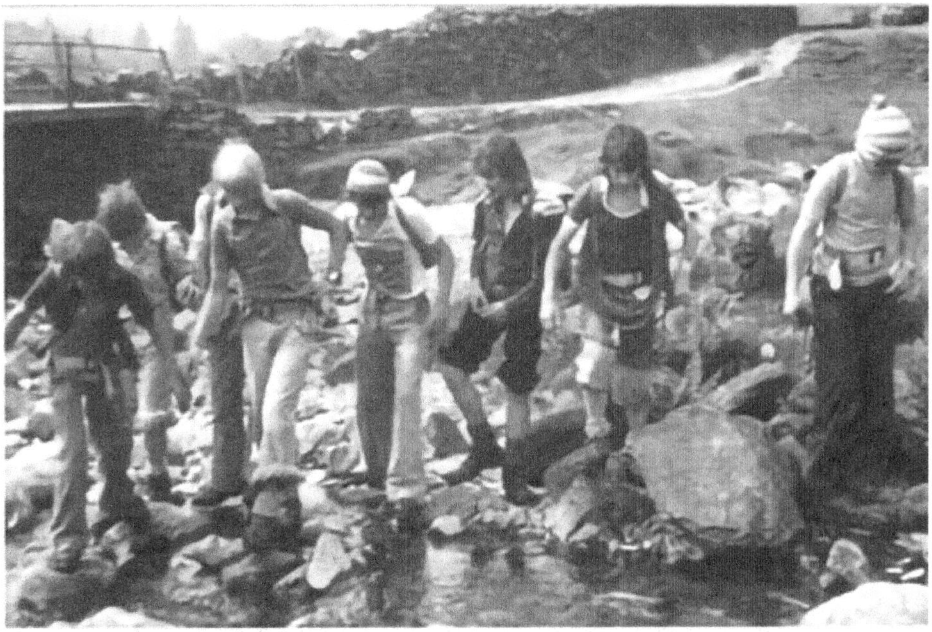

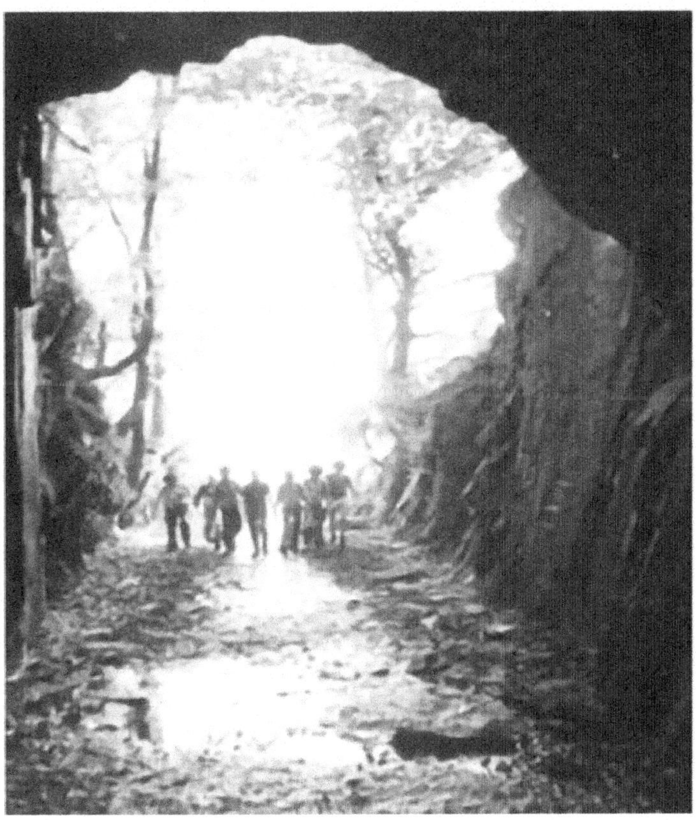

~ THE PIONEERING INSTRUCTORS AND TEACHERS ~

Phil Watkin was one of the founder teachers and provided the following contribution to the pamphlet 'Plas Gwynant: The First 25 Years 1958-1983', which was produced by Sandwell Metropolitan Borough of Sandwell Department of Education.

Phil Watkin, Former Plas Gwynant Teacher

At Plas Gwynant we do not provide schoolchildren with holidays, nor are we attempting to introduce them to activities as a basis for future recreation. We do not even view ourselves as an extension of physical education. We are primarily dedicated to personal and social development in a way in which will be described shortly. In this role, we see ourselves as complementary to a child's normal education in secondary schools.

In the main we run nominal two-week 'adventure courses', a name which is a useful label for school children and schools, but which belies the true nature of the courses. I shall describe these courses in some detail. In addition, we run a number of other courses; one-week 'field study' courses, courses for children of school leaving age and courses for teachers interested in developing an interest in outdoor activities. With the partial exception of the last three days of the course there is no fixed programme of activities for the groups. It is an integral part of the instructor's job to select appropriate activities for his group on a day-to-day basis using whatever criteria he feels appropriate.

There is a wide range of activities from which to choose, from the more glamourous activities of canoeing and abseiling to the more physically demanding activities of map and compass work, orienteering and unaccompanied walks to the more adventurous activities such as coastal exploration, underground exploration, cliff traverses, the ascent of waterfalls, the descent of gorges etc.

On the first day of a course the instructor will usually take his group for a mountain walk, thus affording an excellent opportunity to talk to the group members and to assess them in a wide variety of ways; who are the strongest/weakest at walking/scrambling uphill/downhill, on grass, rocks, over streams, bogs? Who are the most determined, interested and receptive? Who are the biggest moaners, the first to give up? What sort of personalities have they got? What backgrounds? What hopes and aspirations? The catalogue is almost endless. Such a wide-ranging assessment provides the instructor with an excellent basis on which to start selecting activities for subsequent days, and so the day-to-day process of assessment and selection of activities begins. Typically, an instructor might commence with a number of half-day activities in order to learn more about the group and to begin to develop certain initial ideas of development. Rock climbing might be selected because the group showed some initial adeptness at scrambling, abseiling as a means of instilling confidence, a day of exploration might suit a weaker group, a big mountain walk might stretch a stronger group, an unaccompanied walk might consolidate their ability to work together in the absence of an instructor.

Initial success at an activity might be extended by more ambitions days, orienteering to extend map and compass work, a canoe trip down a river or at sea to extend canoeing ability. For some groups, a variety of more generalised activities might be appropriate, with a visit to old mine workings for underground exploration, or scrambling up waterfalls.

For example, although orienteering might be used to knock complacency out of a group who have failed to show they are capable of applying themselves sensibly to these skills; an unaccompanied walk might be used to relieve the tensions between an instructor and a persistently difficult group.

The process only differs toward the end of the course when an overnight camp always takes place and on the final day when the course members are expected to responsibly clean and hand in all their equipment in good order and to undertake a job of some sort which will in some way enhance the Centre or its relationships with the neighbouring communities. The overnight camp in reality comes as an ultimate challenge to the group. Although its timing is not at the discretion of the instructor, its nature and location are. It can vary from a high-level mountain camp or bivouac. Whatever the choice, it will finalise the development of the group and individual which has been the instructor's task throughout the course.

In attempting to achieve personal and social development of the course members, attitudes and behaviour are initial targets for attention. Responsibility, maturity, understanding, tolerance and sympathy are encouraged. Confidence, self-respect and respect for others are instilled. Course members are encouraged to organise themselves individually and as a group. They are helped to come to terms with their own strengths and weaknesses, abilities and limitations. They are helped to face challenges and cope with them at their own level. Their ability to relate to each other and to adults is nurtured. It is our hope that each child will leave Plas Gwynant with a more responsible and mature attitude to life, with increased respect for themselves and others, with increased confidence and a greater ability to face the many problems and challenges with which he will inevitably be faced on leaving school.

It would be wrong to suggest that all these things are achieved with every child passing through Plas Gwynant. Not only does each child and each group start the course at a certain level of development, but each will develop at a rate determined not only by the ingenuity of the instructor but also by the degree of resistance to the process. With some children we may have considerable success and yet feel that we could or should have achieved more. On the other hand, with a particularly perverse child we might congratulate ourselves on some small but significant improvement in attitude. Hopefully we can achieve something with every child and on average sufficient to justify our existence. Occasionally we have to admit failure but more usually we are happy with the results of our efforts. I hasten to add that such results as we do achieve do not stem from the outdoor activities alone, but from the total residential experience.

The problems of living together within the Centre provide yet more valuable challenges for the course members to face, and these can be more difficult to resolve than those of the activities. There is always an instructor on duty to cope with such difficulties that do arise, and the visiting teachers have a large role to play in that respect.

Whilst on the subject of visiting teachers, it is worth mentioning that they too stand to gain considerably from the course as a whole. We frequently find that a suitably receptive teacher develops new and valuable relationships with the children which can bring considerable benefit for long after the course ended. To help them in this process they are encouraged to join in with the group activities alongside the course members. From all that has been said of these 'adventure courses' it might be wrongly assumed that our ideal intake would be entirely 'problem' children. However, although such children may indeed have most to gain from our courses, our success depends at least in part on the society within the Centre, approaching normality. A course made up entirely of 'difficult' children would be very abnormal, as would a single sex course and we have found in the past that such courses can bring almost insuperable problems. However, although we would hope for a reasonably normal cross-section of children, we do expect some bias towards children of lower academic ability, and we certainly do expect at least a normal quota of 'troublemakers'. A more accurate deduction about our ideal intake would be that what we offer has more relevance the closer the children are to leaving school.

Unfortunately, current organisation of schools usually precludes the offering of our courses to fifth years and we must therefore content ourselves with receiving fourth years in the main. Certainly, our ability to have any enduring impact on younger children is doubtful. Besides, both the nature of our established equipment and the demands of the activities give us difficulties in accommodating younger children. Twice a year we run courses for children of school-leaving age. This helps to satisfy two different demands. The first is from children who have otherwise been denied an opportunity to come to Plas Gwynant, possibly because they are more academically able and the pressure of school work on them has been too great. The second demand is from youngsters who through attending our normal 'adventure courses' develop a real interest in one or other of the activities we introduce them to. Having awoken an interest in these youngsters, we have a responsibility to help them develop that interest. Due to the nature of our intake on these courses, they do tend to be run on more recreational lines. And where possible, we help individuals to develop specific skills. Nonetheless, our basic philosophy of personal and social development still underlies everything that we do.

It is one thing to articulate what one is trying to achieve, it is quite another to actually achieve it. Despite 25 years of operation Plas Gwynant is still trying to find ways of getting the most out of its courses. To this end, we try to maintain a healthy discussion of what we are doing. At the end of each course each instructor writes a report in which he attempts to summarise what has been achieved. As a result of this we are regularly analysing our actions and are always receptive to new ideas. In recent months, we have been considering new ways of getting youngsters to become aware of how they are performing. Most recently this has taken the form of a fairly rudimentary self-assessment, the youngsters being asked to give themselves a rating for such things as how they are helping others, or how successful they are being at 'not moaning'. Recently too, we have been having some debate on the way we select the initial groups, since the group composition can itself have a considerable effect on what we are ultimately able to achieve. Another relatively new development has been getting schools to share courses rather than having one school at a time. Despite prophesies of disaster from many schools, this method of operating seems to be beneficial.

Finally, I hope that from what I have said I do not need to emphasise the fact that not only are we not an educational 'frill' but in the present climate of unemployment, financial hardship and social disruption, when school children are questioning the value of the traditional type of schooling, the importance and relevance of the Plas Gwynant experience is increasing all the time.

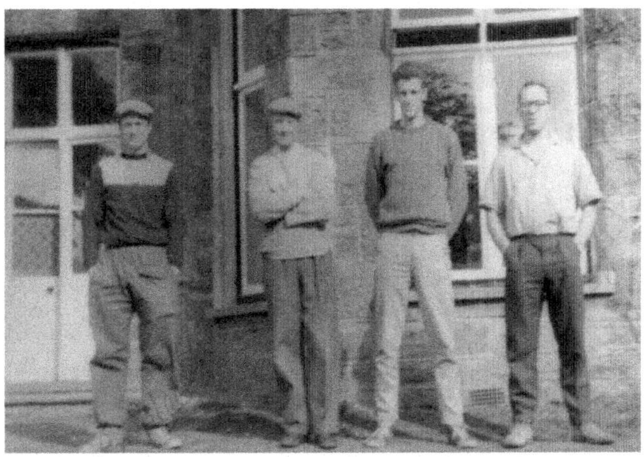

On the left: Murray Watterson

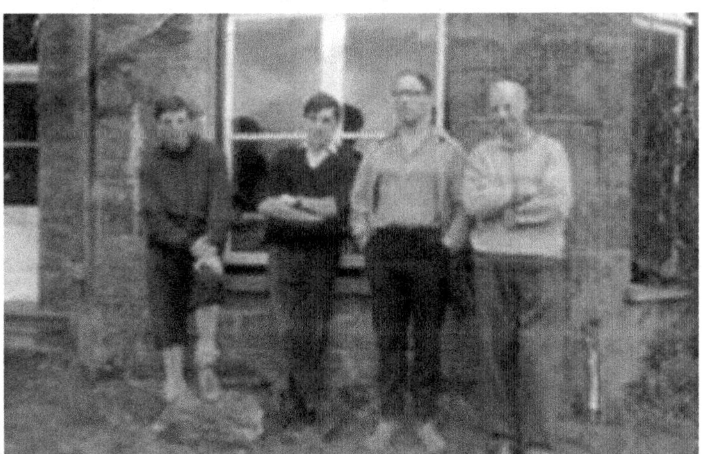

c1965 – L-R: Alan Hole (?), Dave Yates, George Simpkin and George (Scottie) Dwyer, whose son was an active member of the Ogwen Valley Mountain Rescue Team for many years from 1966

George (Scottie) Dwyer had patents for the first climbing nut invented

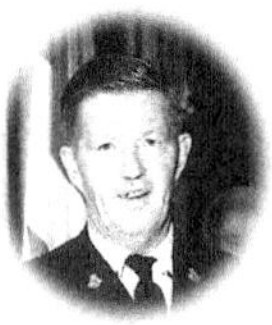

By the early 60's, climbers like John Brailsford saw the commercial potential and developed 'The Acorn', the first climbing nut that was produced and marketed as climbing protection. Brailsford very soon had improved the design and gave the climbing world the legendary Moac. However, evidence unearthed several years ago by North Wales climber Ken Latham, suggests that the modern climbing nut - as we know it - was developed in North Wales as far back as 1946, its inventor being one Scottie Dwyer. A minor figure in the world of North Wales climbing but someone who was responsible for several classic first ascents including one of the regions great VS climbs; the superb 400' mountaineering route, Central Route on Llech Ddu in the Carneddau.

Scottie's Fellow climber Ken Latham shares his memories on how Scottie invented this remarkable piece of equipment

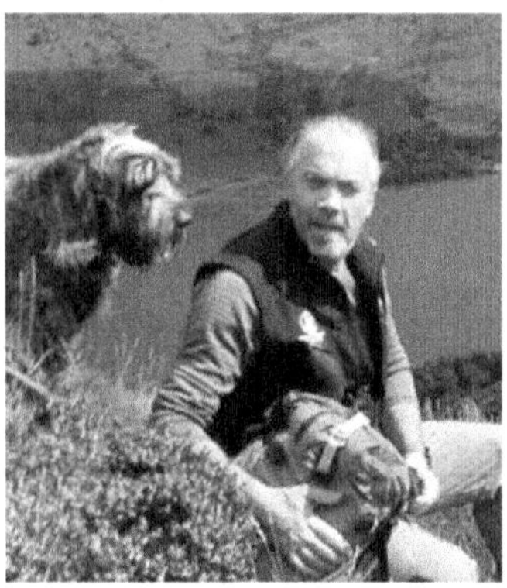

During the summer of 1972, I was managing the Ellis Brigham shop in Capel Curig. On the staff at that time was George 'Scottie' Dwyer. I can't remember now if he was just helping out as a favour, or working there on a regular basis; but from what I recall, he was retired from guiding and just came in to sort out the hire equipment. He hadn't climbed for many years. Indeed, a hip replacement had curtailed his mountaineering activities somewhat (remember in those days, hip jobs really were a bit of a nut and bolt affair).

It was during a quiet day that we got talking. Generally, he kept himself to himself most of the time, so it was a real bonus when he came through to the rear of the shop, carrying a couple of brews and began telling stories of his exploits. Some of the expeditions in the forties and fifties, driving overland to the Himalayas, seemed fantastical; encounters with hoods and bandits were commonplace. He also talked about his climbing in this country and of course, his first ascent of Central Route on Llech Ddu. As the day wore on and Scottie became more forthright, he handed me a metal wedge on a thin piece of line. He seemed to hold back as I examined this crude bit of gear, but asked me for my thoughts about it. I was used to Moac and Clog wedges that were then on the market and I remember being fairly unimpressed at first. It was only a while later that this encounter took on a special significance.

Scottie told me he had been working on some ideas for protection devices for rock-climbing, but did not have the means to get them made up. The nut he showed me was a rough mock-up of one he had made in 1946. I was astounded. He said that he had never used it on a climb and was unsure of its holding properties.

The line available then was hemp and would in all probability not have withstood the stress of a leader fall. Scottie told me he had re-discovered the nut as he was clearing out some old

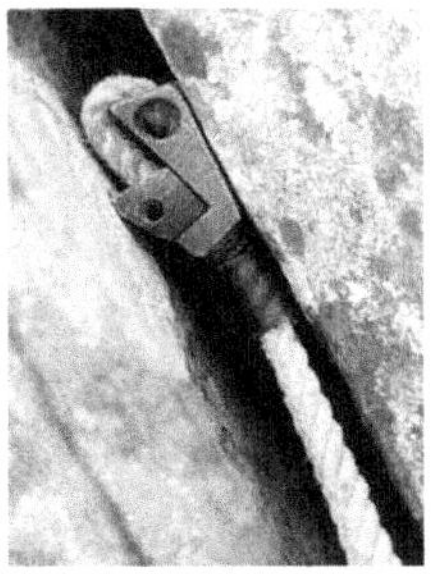

The remarkable 'Scottie' 1946

equipment and had promptly forgotten about it. He asked me to keep it as he had no use for it anymore. I returned to Liverpool and sadly, Scottie died soon after, while still only in his sixties.

Almost 25 years later I was having what everyone will recognise as one of those loft-cleaning sessions in which everything must go, when I came across a long-forgotten sack.
Rummaging through the gear it contained Moacs, Leeper pegs and Peck runners and then I found the 'Scottie' nut. I considered what to do with it. Reluctant to show it around at first, though interested to find if anyone could shed light on other bits of its history, I took it to the CC Centenary Dinner. Many eminent members looked at it, and when they heard its story, commented that it seemed entirely possible it did indeed originate in the year Scottie claimed. It may well be that Scottie couldn't countenance introducing such a piece of equipment in the 1940s; it would no doubt have been seen as unethical. Then he mislaid or forgot about it for years until he told me about it.

If Scottie had found a maker for his nut in the 1940s and launched it on the growing market, who could say how the history of British rock- climbing would read today? The design - combining variable, sliding camming and multi-faceted placement - was at least fifteen years ahead of its time. I showed it to Joe Brown recently and he was convinced of its authenticity; he also commented that he hadn't used any machined nuts himself until about 1961, as he thought they were unethical. Slings on pebbles were still in widespread use.

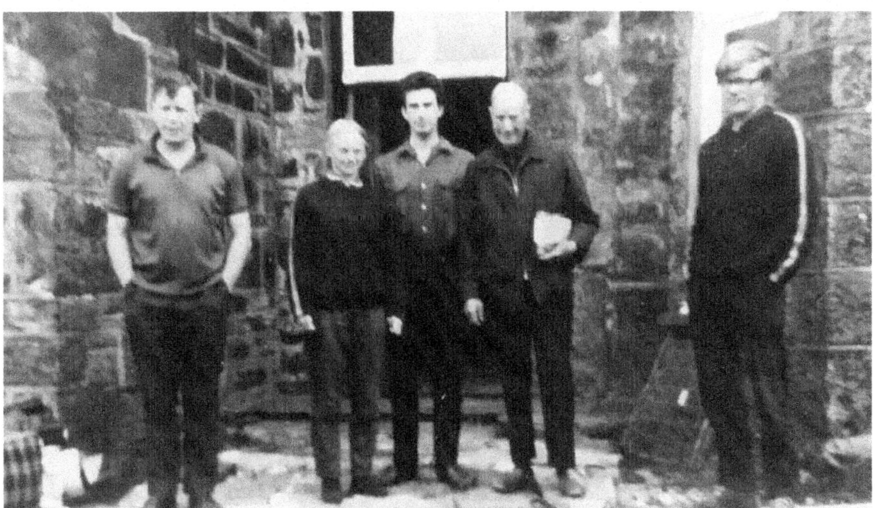

1967, L-R: Murray Watterson, Ruth Townson, John Davidson, George (Scottie) Dwyer and Ian Maxwell

Rosemary Winnall MBE (nee Lillyman) - Memories of Plas Gwynant in the 1970s

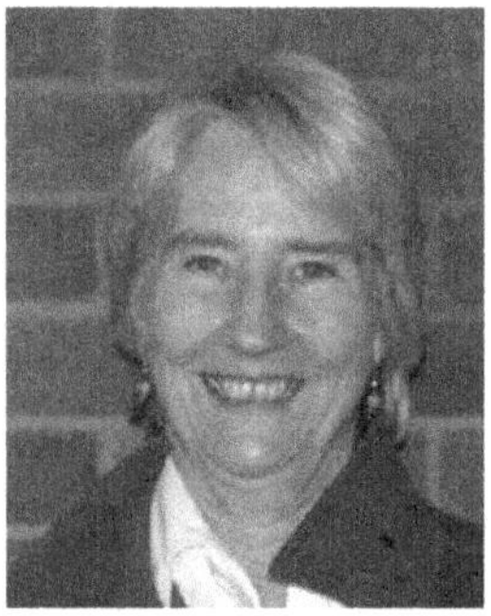

Early in 1970 I was alerted to a staff vacancy at Plas Gwynant by my college biology lecturer Jean Dilnot. She was a member of the Pinnacle Club along with Gwen Moffat and Plas Gwynant staff member Peggy Wild all of whom met regularly at the club hut in Nant Gwynant.

I remember the delight when I heard from centre head Murray Watterson that I had got the job and was to become one of the instructors at this well-known West Bromwich Outdoor Pursuits Centre. But my Principal at Chelsea College of Physical Education was not so happy and called me into her office to tell me how I was wasting 4 years of quality education by taking up the position! Little did she know how valuable I was to find this work with young people, encouraging their personal development and self-esteem.

I had specialised in Outdoor Pursuits at college and I couldn't wait to get into post where Peggy Wild and Nigel Matthews were already working as instructors. Scotty Dwyer was about to retire, and it was a pleasure to meet this Snowdonia Mountain Guide who'd become a legend in his lifetime. Alan Hunt was appointed to replace him and he and I were to work together. I learnt so much from Alan who was a very experienced mountaineer and rock climber, and such a patient leader for the youngsters. In those days 24 students came to stay at the Centre for 3 weeks at a time. They were chosen from several different schools and had no teacher with them, so one of us had to accompany the coach from Beddgelert to West Bromwich to pick them up and return them at the end of the course. Later, students came for 10 days and then we worked straight through followed by 4 days off. We got to know the young people in our care very well and it was great to see their confidence, fitness and self-confidence grow over the time they were with us.

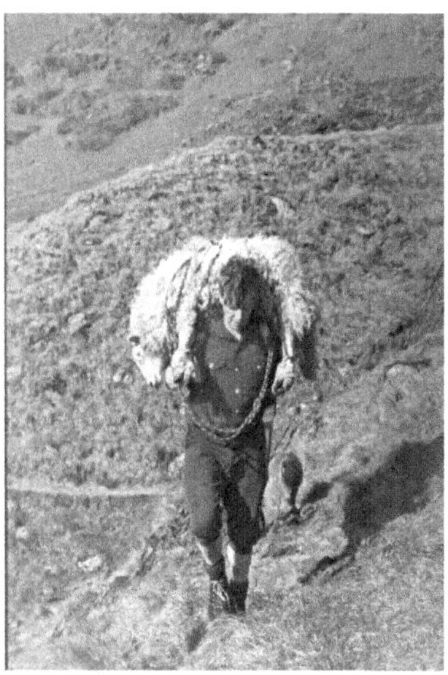

Murray Watterson bringing down an injured sheep, April 1974

During my 4 years at Plas Gwynant I also worked with fellow instructors John Taylor, Clive Hudson, Maggy Willis and Dave Firth and we enjoyed some great times together. We used to organise some exciting days out in our free time and memories include canoeing out to the Skerries off NW Anglesey, climbing Amphitheatre Buttress by moonlight, exploring some of the old abandoned copper mines with ropes and torches, evening climbs at Tremadoc, competing in the first Karrimor Mountain Marathon, and entering local canoe slaloms competitions. Some of us spent holidays together climbing in Chamonix, exploring the Pembrokeshire coast by canoe, mountaineering in Scotland and skiing in the Alps.

Murray Watterson ably led a great team and there was a tradition in those days for all the staff to walk together up Snowdon from Pen y Pass by the light of the harvest moon in September. The kitchen and grounds staff, including Nell, Nancy and Ernie, were not as fit as the instructors, but we all helped each other and everyone succeeded. And this was before the term team-building had been invented!

Occasionally the staff would be called upon by the local farmer to rescue a sheep that was stuck on one of the mountain ledges. Murray was well experienced at this task and directed proceedings when we arrived at the site armed with ropes and a large net. Occasionally the animal was injured or very weak and had to be carried down the mountain.

Our staff duty day started with a long drive in the Land Rover to pick up Nell Dwyer our cook (Scotty's wife) at 7.00am from her mountain cottage, situated up a steep drive on the side of the Glyders. I remember that this was not too much fun in the depths of winter, but the vehicle had 4 wheel drive and I soon became competent at operating this and double-declutching. The domestic duties rota for the course participants was a major part of their social training whilst they were with us, and we had to supervise bed making, cleaning and washing up before morning inspection by Murray.

Memories of activities with the children include abseiling down Eagle Rock, climbing on Gladstone Rock, canoe surfing at Black Rock Sands, orienteering by canoe on Llyn Gwynant, exploring the copper mine and finding fool's gold, and camping out up in the hills. Occasionally in the winter I would take a group beach-combing for the day on Llanddwyn Island on Anglesey, or we would visit the Hairy Man's Cave on the side of Lliwedd.

In the evenings I particularly remember singing songs around the campfire, and encouraging the children to write poetry. But it was the mountaineering that stood out – encouraging the youngsters to get to the top, and sharing their exhilaration when they succeeded.

Rags the terrier belonged to Murray and Beryl Watterson and she always wanted to come with us on our walks. She would join us in all seasons, and in bad weather sometimes had to be carried home in a rucksack especially when her hair became frozen making it impossible for her to see!

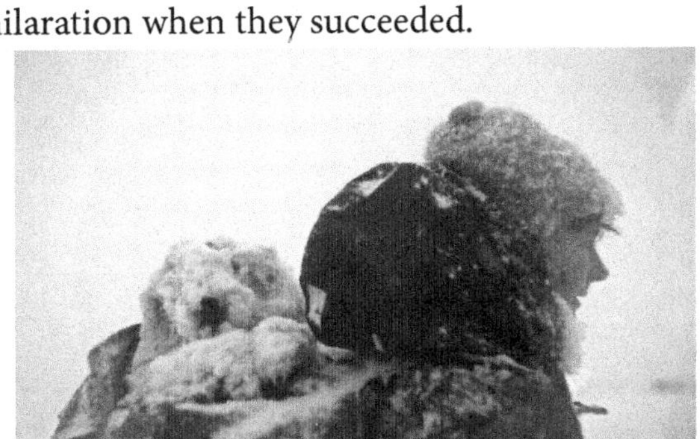

Rags the terrier carried by Peggy Wild, January 1974, coming down from Snowdon

The children related well to this little dog that did so much to encourage the shy and comfort the homesick. Wilbur the cat adopted me soon after I arrived probably because she found a way to climb up and into my bedroom where she slept each night.

I left Plas Gwynant in 1974 to run Rhossili Outdoor Pursuits Centre for West Glamorgan LEA, but I was invited to join the Plas Gwynant Expedition to Iceland as one of the leaders in the summer of 1975. Clive Hudson was our excellent expedition organiser and we took with us older students who'd been to Plas Gwynant from Dartmouth High School and Wodensborough Youth Centre. This was a special 3 weeks when all the training in Snowdonia was essential for us to successfully carry out a reconnaissance survey of the glaciers in Central Trollaskagi in connection with the Young Explorers Trust project on glacier retreat. No-one used the term climate change in those days! This was a very successful expedition leading to life-long friendships.

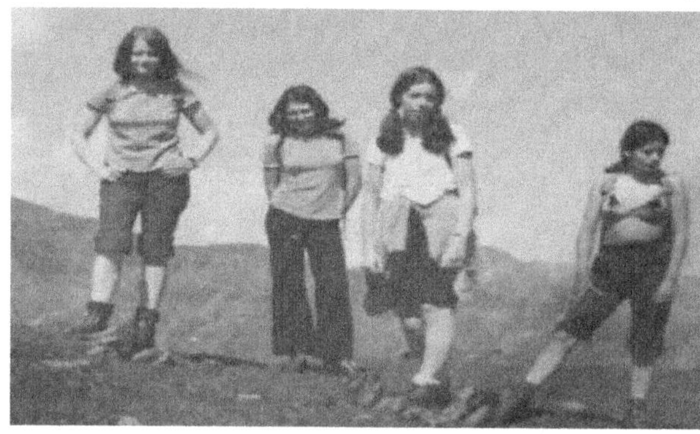

Rosemary's photograph of a group of girls on Yr Aran, early 1970s

I have many happy memories of my time at Plas Gwynant and I am so glad to know that young people are still able to benefit from the experience. Below are two of several poems I've kept from students in the 1970s.

PLAS GWYNANT
by Gary Gibbs (aged 14)
from Woodgreen High School

Deep in Wales, by the hills,
West Bromwich kids go for thrills.
In the valley by the mountains,
Nearby the lakes and fountains.
Plas Gwynant is the houses's name,
A picture good enough to frame.
Up the mountains in the lake,
Our backs very nearly break.
Plas Gwynant is the place to be,
At least it is the place for me.

MIST
by Teresa Predota (aged 15)
from Menzies High School

It came; Tumbling, erupting out of nothing
Across the dull grey sky.
Neutral and moisture-filled,
Shifting and rolling,
Rippling into fingers and tendrils,
Slithering to and fro.
Meeting, separating, cooling,
Melting into other mists and clouds;
Broken by the wind and sun, it dissolves,
To form another mist;
It goes. Destroyed and absorbed by the sun's warmth
It evaporates and slowly wisps away;
It trails and disappears, Yet to come again.

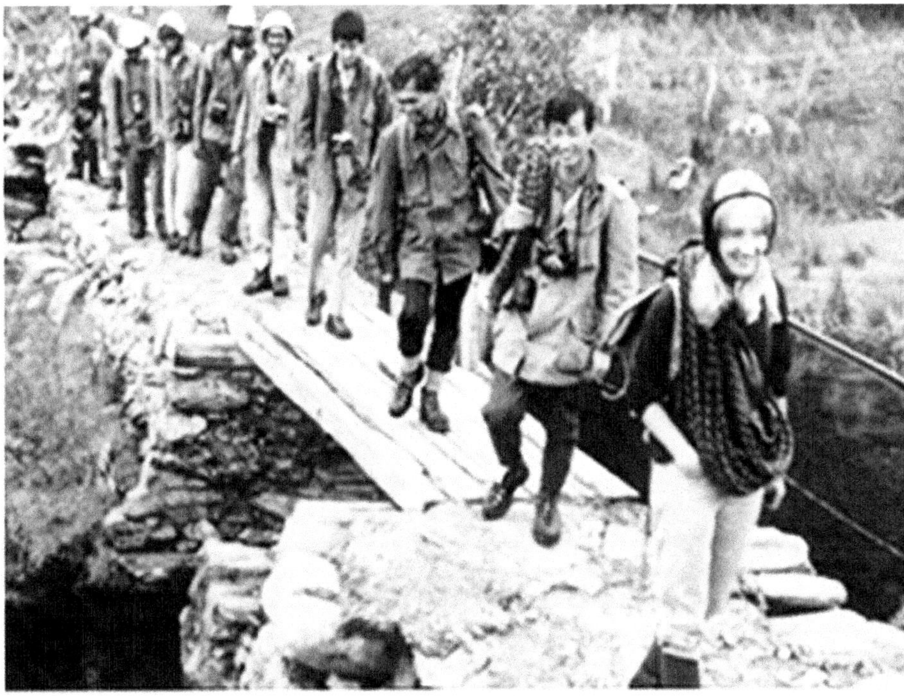

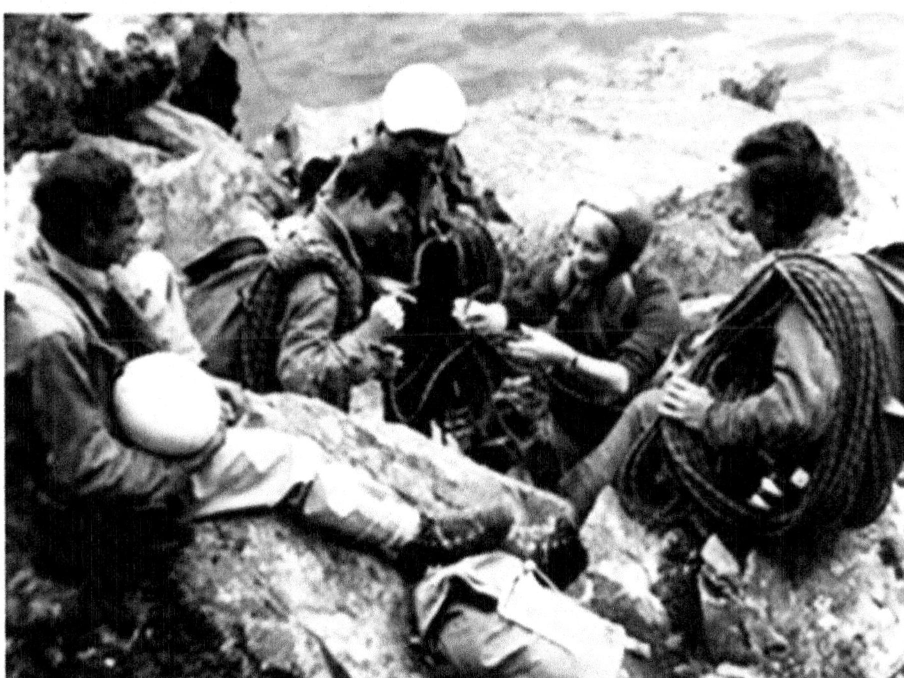

Rosemary leading members of a photography course early 1970s

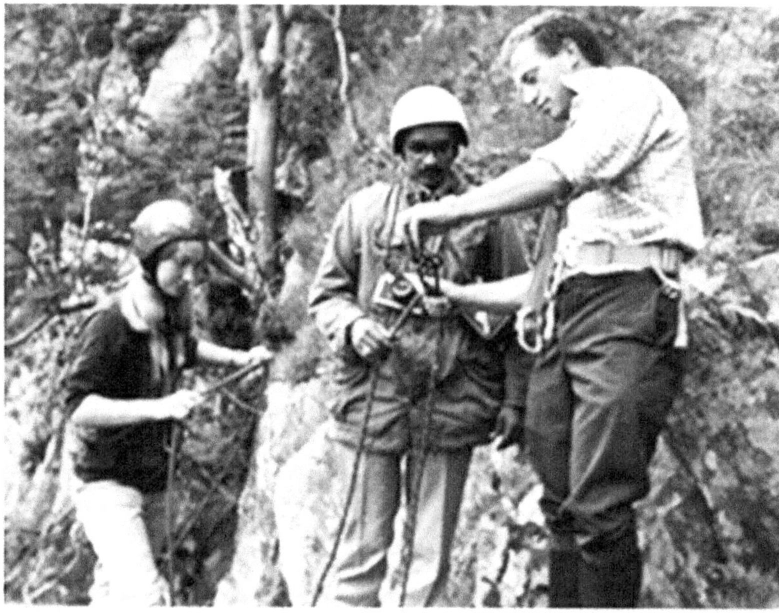

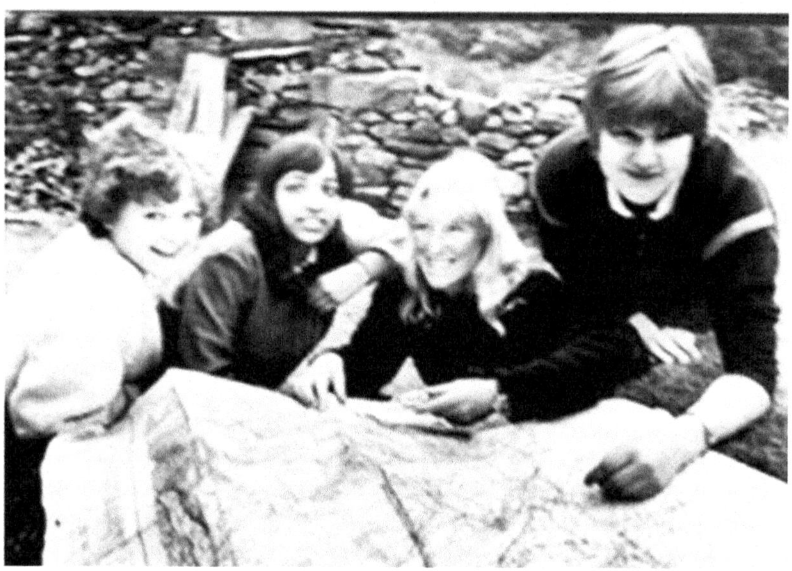

Rosemary map reading with students circa 1970s

Rosemary later moved on to work as an Education Manager for the Forestry Commission in Wyre Forest and is a founder member of the Wyre Forest Study Group, committee member of Worcestershire Recorders and a keen wildlife photographer. She also started the Wyre Forest Discovery Centre, which she ran for 13 years before retiring. For services to the natural environment for her work as a volunteer to champion the Wyre Forest, Rosemary received an MBE in 2015.

Clive Hudson, former Tutor at Plas Gwynant 1971-1986

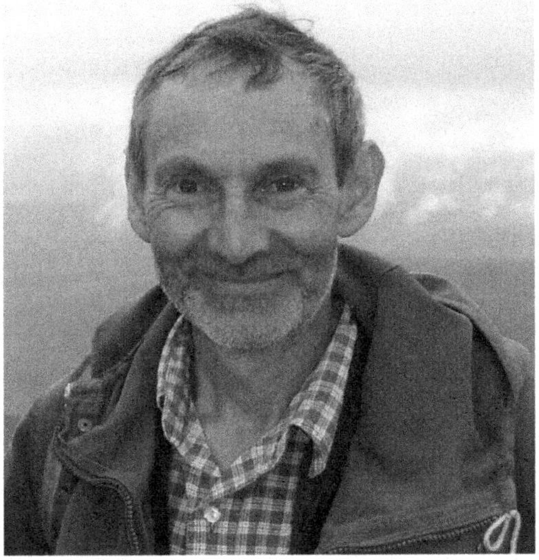

My Very Happy Memories!

When I got the job of Instructor at Plas Gwynant, I thought I had got the Best Job Ever; I had! My own Secondary Modern schooling was not ferociously academic, but by luck of circumstances I discovered geology and my world vision exploded! Teacher training and a degree followed, and all these life experiences forged a passion to inspire young people to the excitement of learning about the beauty of the Natural World that I had been very lucky to stumble into. Along the way I had Youth Hostelling holidays in the Lake District, leading to a thirst to engage with the exciting skills of mountaineering, rock climbing, and canoeing. Working at Plas Gwynant (PG) was an amazing opportunity to engage and share these passions working with pupils both on Adventure and Field Study Courses.

For two years I worked alongside Rosemary Winnall (née Lillyman), John Taylor and Peggy Wild, under the Warden Murray Watterson. Space is limited so I will add my own pot-pourri of memories of contemporary staff, the educational thinking for the existence of Plas and a tiny selection of memorable events out of, maybe, 400 courses that I must have experienced!

As a trained teacher I wanted to complete my Probationary Year. Previously the administration had differed and this 'completion' been granted 'on the job', or had not been relevant to staff members. A new Education Inspector insisted I should be seen in a 'class-room situation' – and no appeal from Murray or me could alter this. The upshot of this was my resigning from Plas Gwynant and then teaching geography and geology at Dartmouth High School under the charismatic Head of Department, John Shobbrook. But change was in the air; 1974 brought the Metropolitan Borough of Sandwell into being and the expansion of Plas from 24 to 40 places and from 4 to 6 staff, plus the Head. As much as I enjoyed my bedsit year in Edgbaston, it was not for me, and I was soon successfully reapplying and getting back to there! Soon after I gained the new post of Deputy Headmaster and so it remained until I resigned in 1986, to create a new life with my wife, building our own home and having children. It has not occurred to me before but my three applications for posts at Plas and my two resignations might be something of a record!

The different titles of establishment and employees are quite revealing. I was first employed as an Instructor at Plas Gwynant Adventure School; the evocative name written on the doors of the Landrover, and Murray was a Warden. Around 1974 the titles changed; the establishment became a Centre for Outdoor Education, we became Teachers of Outdoor Education, and Murray became a Headmaster. The courses were also changing; the pre-breakfast immersion in the pool at the bottom of the falls in the Afon Llyn Edno (for duty staff as well as pupils!), the tree felling (with axes) seen in a black and white film made to record the first course, and the general 'hardness' of the courses was amended for all youngsters, and not just the most physically able. Although Murray certainly had a disciplinarian side to him, he had after all been an Army Physical Training Instructor; he had a clear vision for a different approach. The activities – mountain walking, climbing, canoeing, camping - were great, but the educational context was the absolute key to more profound learning experiences, and indeed, the justification for the existence of the establishment itself. This extra context was visualised and developed by Murray.

I am now reflecting on memories that are over 3 decades ago (gulp!), and my thoughts about Plas may be seen as viewed through rainbow tinted lenses. But I have always believed that the Adventure Courses had two huge educational Foundation stones; firstly, the length of the Course; and, secondly, the continuity of the staff member with each group. The twelve day Course, the reduction from the original three week course, gave ten full activity days, and the contact time with one member of staff was equivalent to approximately a year of classroom teaching. The 'group' - including the same staff member - was so important. A youngster may be able to demonstrate a 'good' or 'naughty' side for two or three days; but after that it is not so easy! As the days go by all the members of the group start to learn a lot about each other, and through all the activities and social dynamics within the group, opportunities arise to nudge against antisocial behaviour and celebrate and encourage good behaviour. This is a huge topic, but it is so important, and should form a fundamental reason for quality outdoor education centres.

To the best of my knowledge this important combination of Adventure Course length and staff/group continuity was unique to Plas and was maintained by Murray for my fifteen year involvement. Oh yes, at times his strictures could irritate! But the Team he assembled and the educational structure and atmosphere he developed gets my applause. His OBE for Services to Education was appropriate. After getting a Deputy, Murray spent more time away from the Centre, particularly in his role as Chair of the Wardens of Mountain Centres, and giving talks at various conferences. He also spent time and energy promoting the Centre and its work within the Education Department and among relevant Borough Councillors. In my early days as an instructor I did sometimes wonder why the boss of the Centre was not out 'in the weather with the rest of us'; I came to realise that 'The Wider Team' for an Outdoor Education Centre includes the administrators and policy-makers who must 'believe' in the value of the work to provide the necessary funding and recourses. Bells may ring at what I have said because many Local Authority outdoor centres have now closed.

With the increase in staff numbers to six, and staff changes over the years, the roll of staff names increased: Maggie Willis, David Firth, Mike Garside, Phil Watkin, Helena Burrows (née Hall), Liz Haynes (née Olerenshaw), Dodi Palmer, Debs McKewon, Derek Weaver. My praise and admiration for all the members of staff I worked alongside at Plas Gwynant is immense. All were totally professional, hardworking, reliable, knowledgeable, excellent with children; oh dear, the list of attributes could, in sincere honesty, go on and on. Just great work mates and friends. As Rosemary has recorded, we had a lot of outdoor adventures together in our own time; this applies particularly in my earlier singleton years. The 'longest day of my life' with John – a 19 hour traverse of Mont Blanc via the Brenva Spur; experiencing the 'strongest wind of my life' with Phil as we battled from the Briaiach, after a night in a snow hole near this Cairngorm summit; and lots, lots more adventures. How very lucky to have such skilled and reliable companions.

I am aware that I have hardly mentioned the Adventure Course (or Field study) activities. Activities and events- memories, memories – Oh I wish there was more space - the time I was 'told off' by the police for going direct to RAF valley and calling out a helicopter; a moment of panic while my group of youngsters were soundly asleep deep inside the Croesor Mine; an unconscious lad near the summit of Snowdon as the darkness loomed and the snow storm intensified...stories, stories...

Rosemary mentioned the Iceland Expedition I organised in 1975 had led to 'life-long relationships'. Out of the 4 staff members there followed one marriage, and out of the 10 youngsters two further marriages. And while on the theme of Plas Gwynant and marriages, I ought to mention Shân my wife, a Welsh girl by name and birth. The connection to Plas Gwynant? Coincidently Shân did her teacher training in the West Midlands, taught at a Sandwell school, and came to Plas as a visiting member of staff. The rest, they say is history; all part of the Plas Gwynant Story!

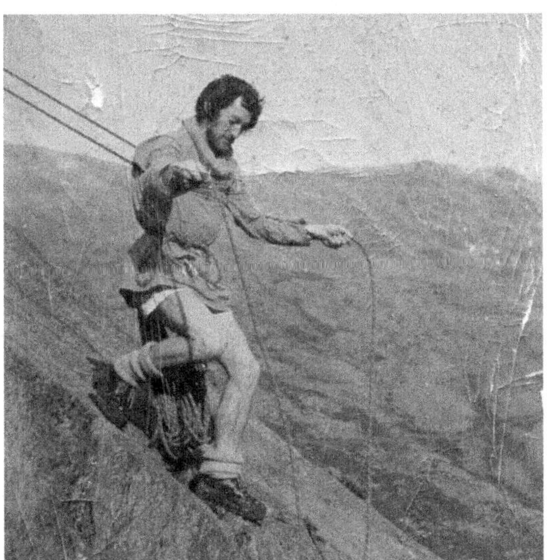

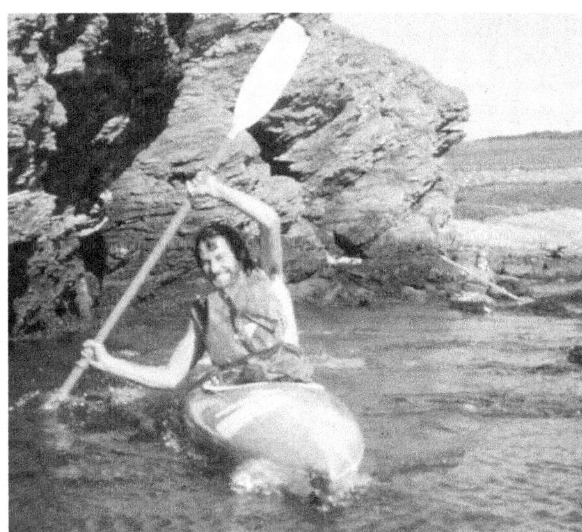

Staff Photographs - courtesy of John Murden - Circa 1990's

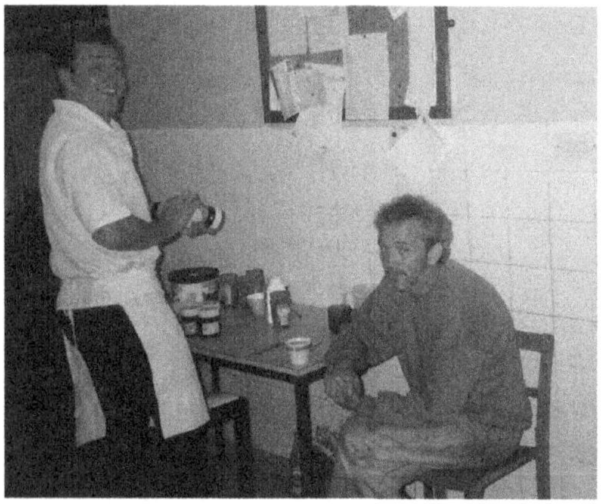

Steve Chapman - cook and Emrys - handyman 1993

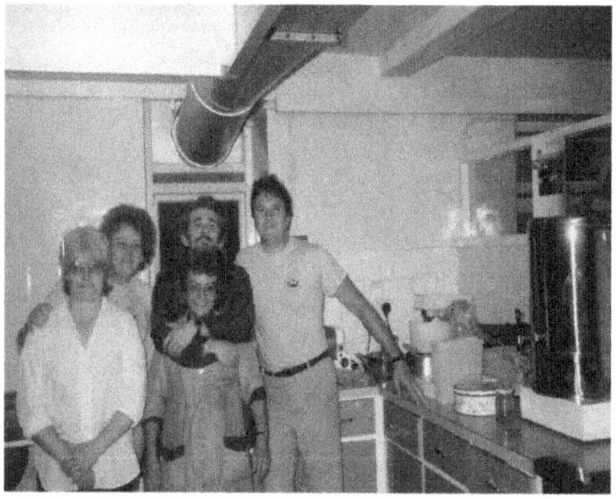

Kitchen staff

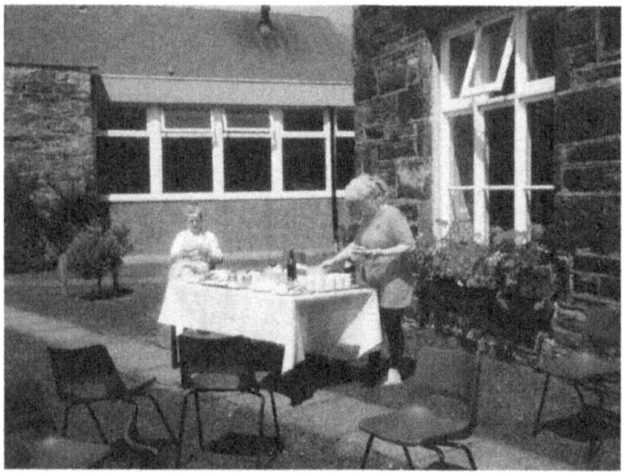

An outdoor meal – Pat Crammer

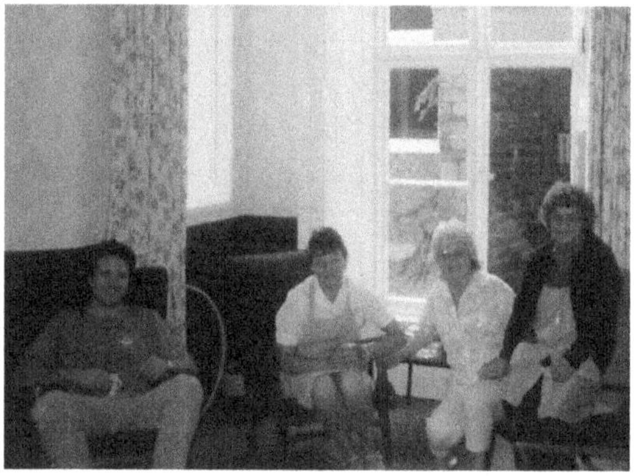

The people behind the scenes

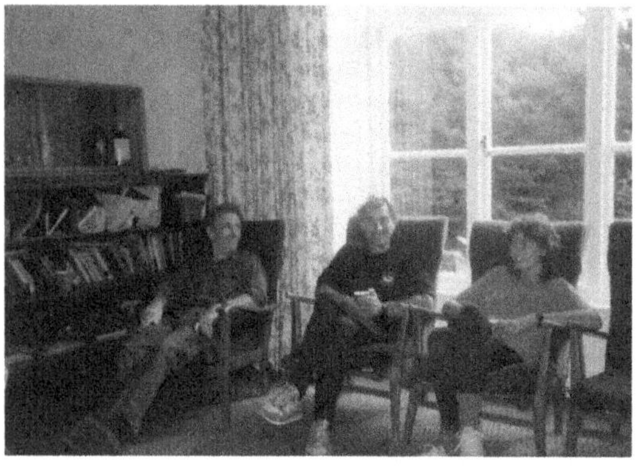

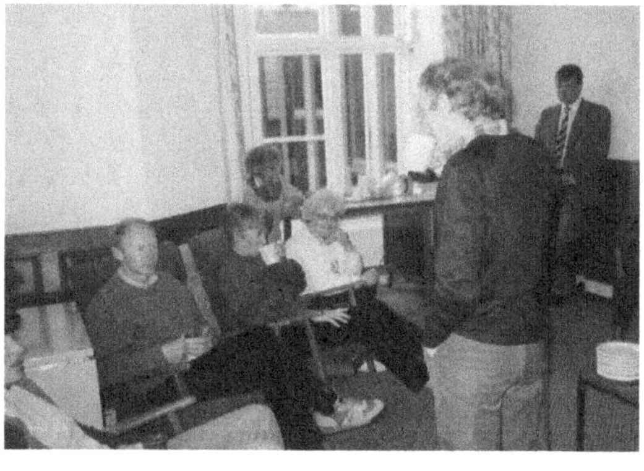

In the staff room – 1993

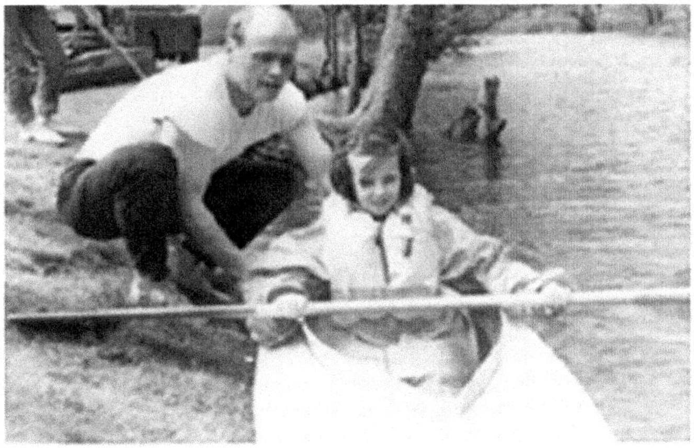

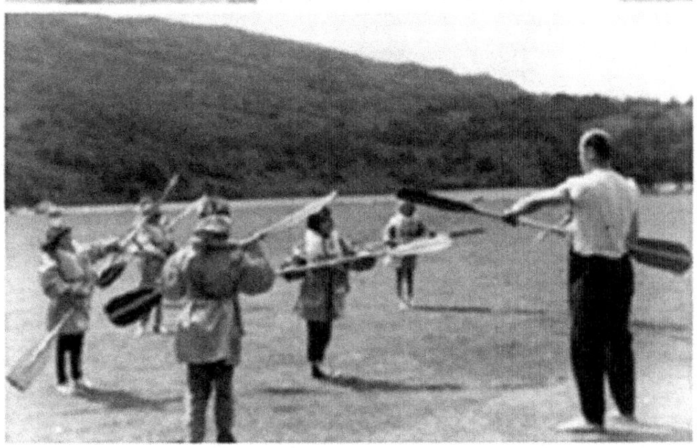

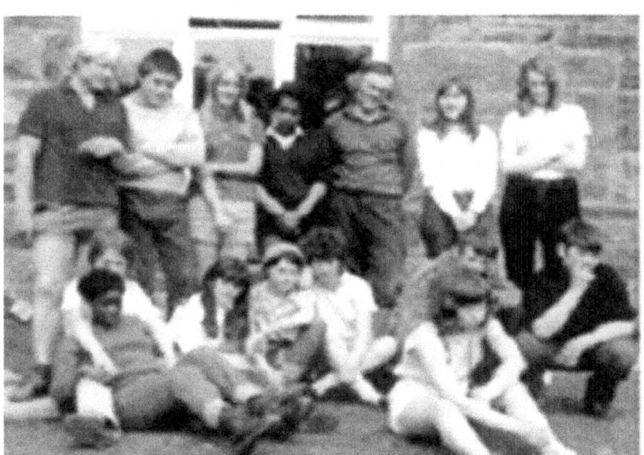

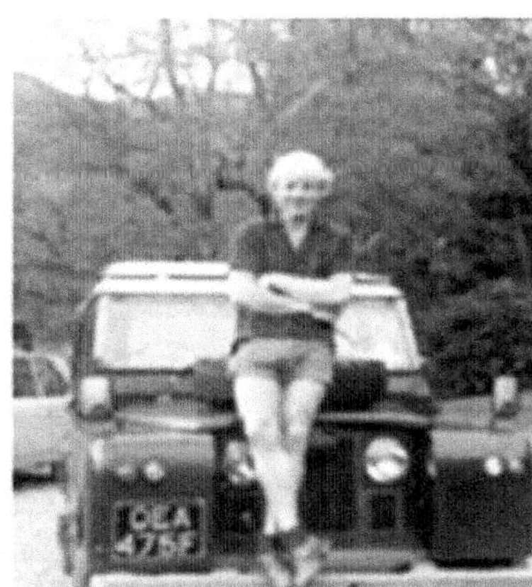

Martin Endicote pictured with students and with his Land Rover

~ PLAS GWYNANT MILLENNIUM PROJECT~

In the year 2000 facilities at Plas Gwynant underwent extensive development, mainly around capacity, heating and disabled access. All of which would herald a new era of larger courses held in a modernised centre, now fit for the new century.

The Plas Gwynant Millennium Development Opening Ceremony was held on 2nd March 2000, by Lord King. His opening speech was recorded:

> Mr Mayor, Members of Sandwell Council, colleagues and friends of Plas Gwynant, It gives me great pleasure to be with you at Plas Gwynant today on the opening of the Millennium Development.
>
> As Leader of the Council and member of the Residential Centres Steering Group, I am particularly proud to have played a part in the modernisation of the Centre and to also have supported the rest of Sandwell Residential Education Service which, through the other three centres of which I am equally proud, has contributed so much to the personal development of thousands of young – and now not so young – people of Sandwell.
>
> I have long held a personal commitment to the service as I have recognised that it is too easy for those amongst us who are able to have access to the countryside to take it for granted. Facilities like Plas Gwynant give Sandwell children and young people a real opportunity to experience a different environment and, through that, to develop as individuals and as citizens of the wider world.
>
> The support of the local community here in North Wales has played an important part in the development of thousands of youngsters from Sandwell schools. This is something we are very conscious of and it is very much appreciated.
>
> The improvements you will see today are the result of many months of hard work by elected members, officers and external partners. As you will see shortly there is still some work for us to do but I am sure that you will agree that we have already been able to carry out a significant amount of work to improve sleeping accommodation, access for the disabled and perhaps most importantly to those in the dormitories, central heating! Firstly, it gives me great personal pleasure, on behalf of the Members of Sandwell Council and the citizens of the Borough to declare the Millennium Development at Plas Gwynant officially OPEN.

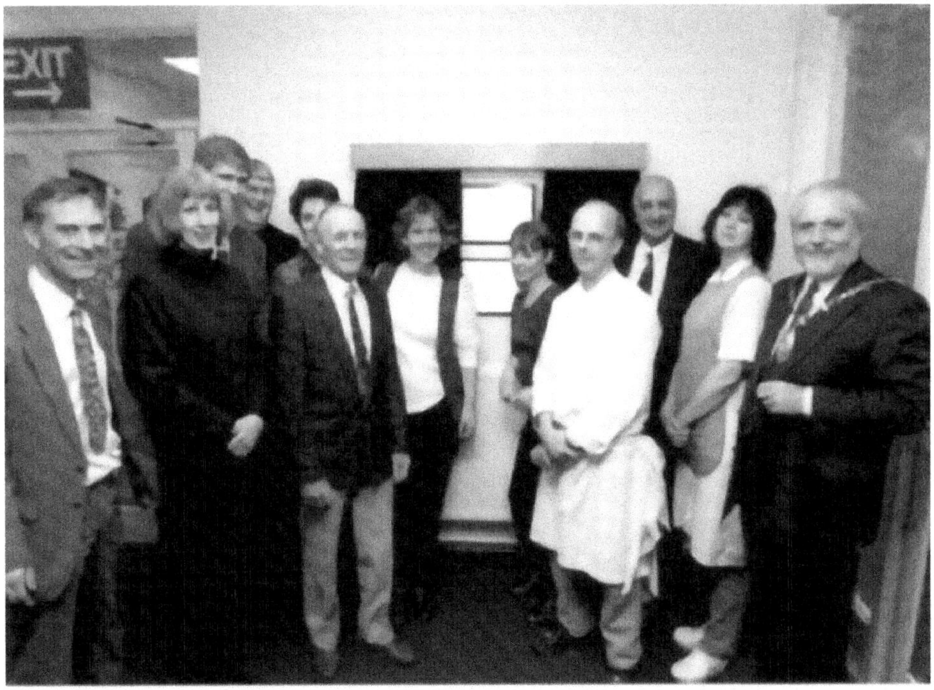

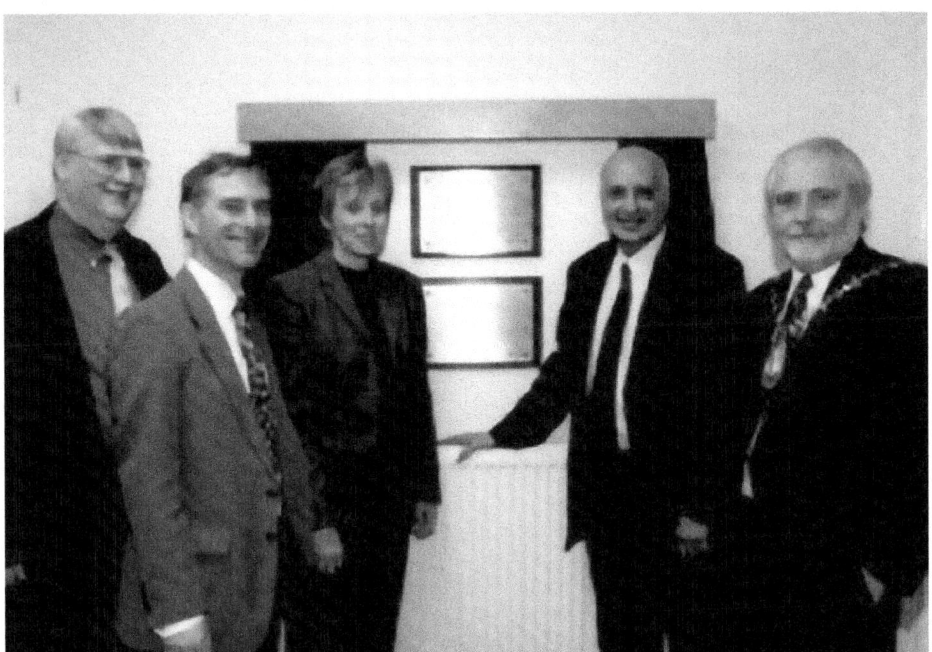

Lord King with Staff and Council members, who attended the unveiling of two plaques,which mark the occasion of the Plas Gwynant Millennium Development Opening Ceremony

~ PLAS GWYNANT REVISITED ~

For several years, former pupils from Sandwell schools have attended an annual weekend reunion at Plas Gwynant. The age range criteria was for those who attended during the 1950s, 60s or 70s. It was a small group at first, but has grown in popularity over the years. Some members attended Plas Gwynant from school when there was no electricity, heating or hot water, yet still remember their experience with great affection and enjoy their reunion weekends every year.

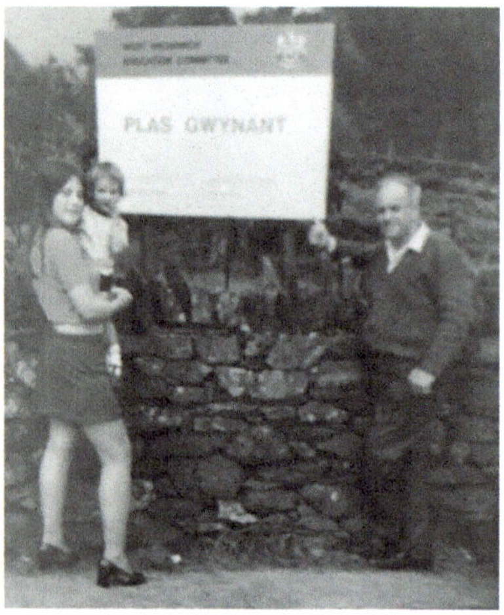

For some, the memories may be simply getting out of the car for a quick photograph, when passing the centre on the way to the coast with our children. Pictured left is Jan Drury with her father, Fred and nephew Tony, doing just that in 1972.

Walter (Wally) Gough attended the very first course in 1958 and confesses he would have loved to have pursued outdoor activities as a career, having excelled in all physical training at secondary school. However, opportunities were limited, so he had to confine his love of the great outdoors to his spare time. Wally also attends the annual reunion weekends without fail, extending his holiday in and around North Wales in his camper van when the weekenders had gone home.

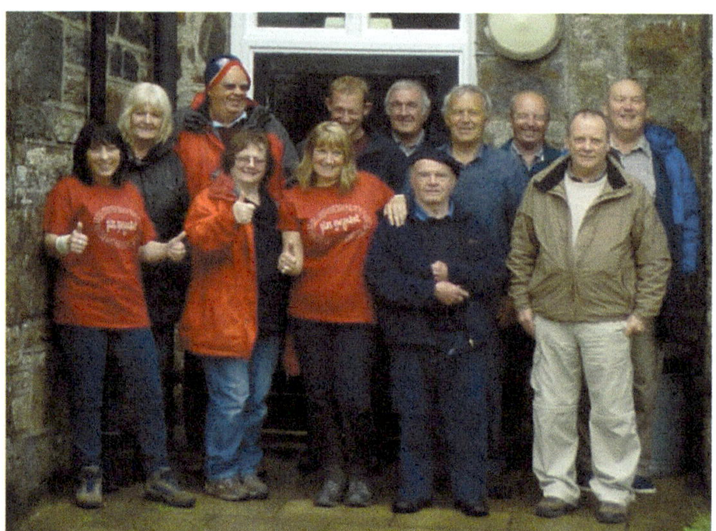

Some members return to the Plas Gwynant reunion every year to try something challenging, like hiking, abseiling, gorge scrambling, canoeing along the Menai Straits and defying 'The Swellies', tackling an underground slate mine, or perhaps to just enjoy the good company, fresh air and outstanding home cooking. Whatever the reason, everyone has a memorable time.

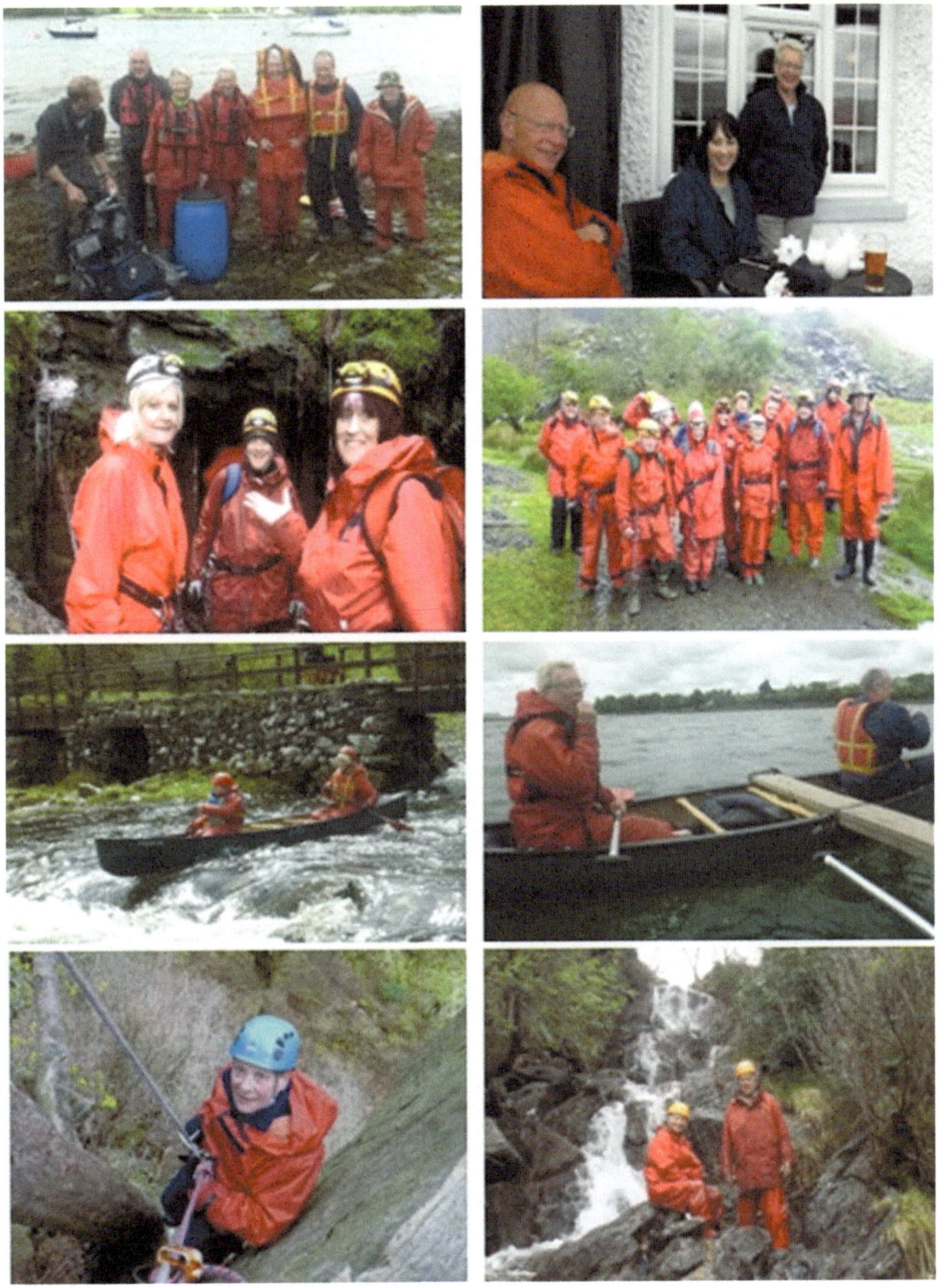

Diehard enthusiasts include Royston Simms, Sue Clarke, Judith Rogers, Gwyneth Hull, Jan Drury, Lynn Woodward, Olwyn Bailey, Stephen Edwards, Ken Lewis, Bill Hall, Derrick Lees, Roger Whitlock, Chris Martin, Gary Rushton, Michael Maher, Wally Gough, Frank Batchelor, Sandra Meredith and many others over the recent years.

~ PLAS GWYNANT TODAY AND TOMORROW~

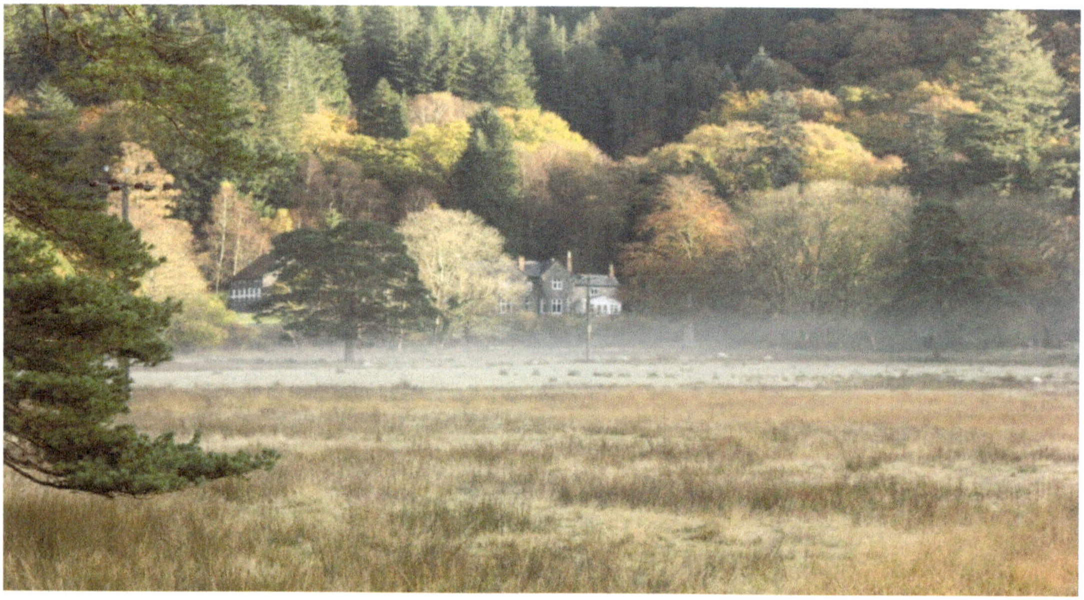

Photograph by Peter Wharton

Richard Oakes, Manager of Residential Education Service, Sandwell MBC

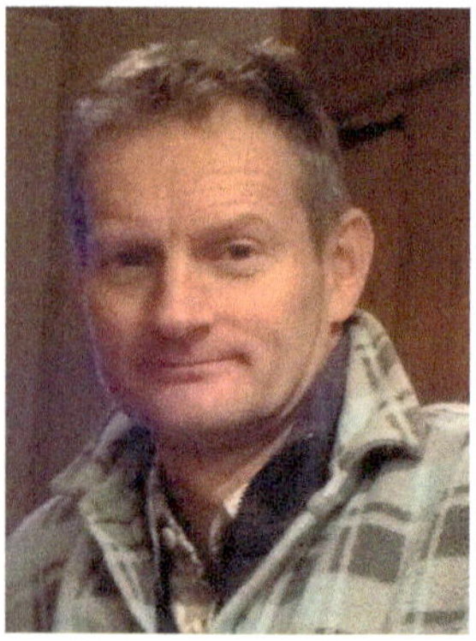

Plas Gwynant is one of four residential education centres proudly owned and run by Sandwell Council as the Residential Education Service. Between them, the centres offer a wide range of settings and activities for experiential learning, with a clear focus on maximizing the opportunities available for Sandwell children and groups. Environmental programmes, forest-based learning, themed courses, and creative arts are all available.

Plas Gwynant, with its dramatic location, sits right at the adventurous end of the scale – what an awesome place for children to visit! Mountains, gorges, lakes, waterfalls, mines, the beach; Plas Gwynant, and its expert team of staff, make real-life learning adventures for visitors which not only develop a wealth of personal and social skills, but offer challenge and discovery that are remembered for a lifetime. The success and reputation of Plas Gwynant is also built on its warm welcome – a sense of being 'home' to those who stay there and, in many ways, to those who work there alongside visitors. Sandwell Council recognises that its centres are probably needed more now than ever before, to develop life skills, academic progress, physical and mental health and to broaden experience and aspirations. Recent investment to upgrade Plas Gwynant is a sign of intent; we are well on track with our plan to ensure that the centres remain accessible and affordable for the future.

Jeff Handley, Head of Plas Gwynant Outdoor Education Centre

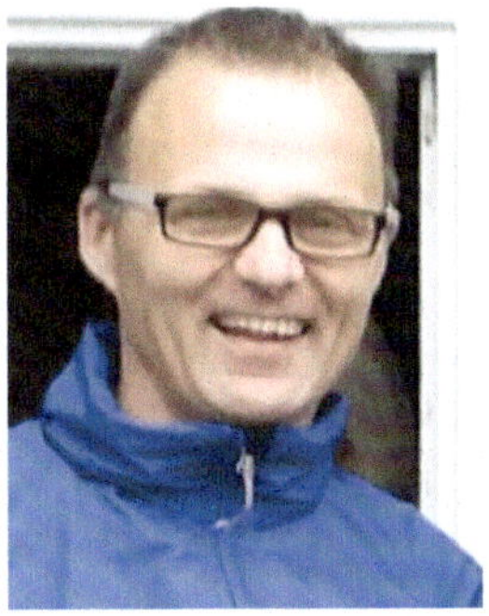

What next for Plas Gwynant?

When I started as Head of Centre at Plas Gwynant in 2005 the world looked very different and I don't think anyone could have predicted the near future. Britain and the world soon had a financial crisis and were in recession, as a result of this long term austerity measures and continuing 'efficiencies' became the norm with the government making their savings from Local Authority spending.

I used to crystal ball gaze and worked with short medium and long term business targets and plans. I liked the certainty of a predictable future, but working closely with the Council and similar organisations, it was obvious that this approach just wouldn't work anymore. The challenge was to make sure we developed a series of options that allowed us to positively, creatively and flexibly respond to changes in the world around us that influenced us, in short we needed to act much more like a business.

Sandwell, as a very forward thinking Local Authority, have been very positive and pragmatic working with us and Sandwell's Residential Service as a whole to ensure the future viability of both Plas Gwynant and the Residential Service. The easy option would have been to close the centre, as many Local Authorities have, however it is recognised that we provide opportunities for the young people of Sandwell that would quickly disappear without our existence. Instead of closure, capital was invested in the building and infrastructure so that we could eventually become cost neutral and as such, provide an education service with no cost to the Council or its tax payers. The capital work was completed in 2017 and we are now moving towards breaking even financially. Sandwell Metropolitan Borough Council clearly sees the value we add to young people and the potential we have to support their wider needs.

The business plan is to have increased use of the centre, this has been made possible by having the centre updated, the accommodation made more flexible and appealing. To make residential trips financially possible for Sandwell children, their families and schools we offset the cost of their courses against courses for non-Sandwell schools that aim to make 'profit'. The increased occupancy has meant that we can do this whilst still having the same amount of Sandwell children visit Plas Gwynant.

Schools come in all shapes and sizes today and despite how they are governed or where they are, their common thread is that they are measured against a set of attainment standards they have to deliver with increasingly shrinking budgets. As a centre we ensure we work very closely with our users to deliver bespoke courses that meet their individual learning needs. What seems to have taken a back seat in schools is personal growth, inspiration, significant new experiences and developing a strong set of values; residential courses used to focus on this, unfortunately schools can no longer justify these key experiences for young people by themselves as they are not visibly measured. To ensure we maximise developmental opportunities on our residential courses we build the above mentioned values into every course as a key entitlement that runs alongside the school's required identified measured outcomes.

So……where next?
I am not sure survival is enough. We need focus, without which no good can be done. Once we can demonstrate we can survive, or rather be cost neutral, we can start looking at how we can make it easier for Sandwell young people to access our service, how we can support Sandwell families and look at the support we can offer those entering employment.

As Head of Centre, my tenure has been and continues to be an interesting journey. At the heart of it is making sure as many young people as possible have the opportunity to experience what I believe is an essential opportunity for personal growth in an inspirational setting. I am proud of what I do and look forwards the future, wherever that journey takes us.

Dan Jackson, Senior Tutor at Plas Gwynant Outdoor Education Centre

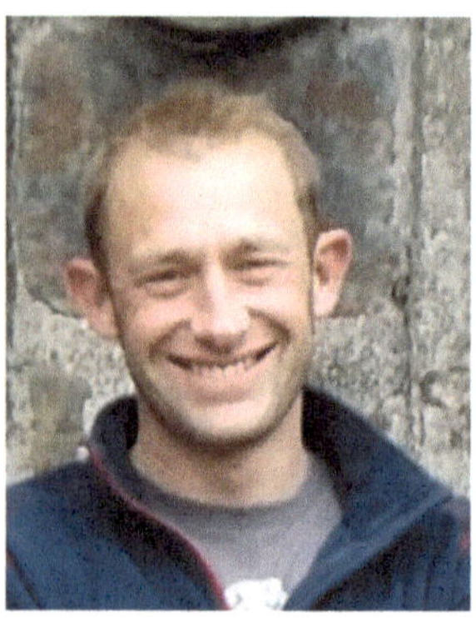

Plas Gwynant today…. Plas Gwynant tomorrow?

If it were possible to plot the historical course of local authority outdoor education centres in the form of a graph, one would create a profile akin to the mountains within which they nestle. A rising and falling line; sometimes gently and sometimes sharply. Ridges and slopes, high peaks and deep valleys. There have been high times and there have been low times. Plas Gwynant's trajectory has been the same as that of any Local Education Authority owned centre and in a world of cuts, deadlines, necessity and efficiency it is a testament to Sandwell Council that there is still an outdoor service to call its own. Outdoor education has never been a compulsory provision for schools within the UK. Successive governments have recognised the enormous benefits that learning outside the classroom brings. However, that measurable link between attainment in school and outdoor learning still evades discovery. Consequently, there is always that underlying worry that lean times will lead to closures and the end of the adventure. The last ten years since the financial crash have seen authorities such as Birmingham, Walsall, Bedfordshire and Worcestershire shedding their residential centres in North Wales and giving them over to the private sector. One, Aberglaslyn Hall, which once belonging to Leicestershire Council and not 5 minutes up the road from Plas Gwynant, now stands empty and in slow decline.

National finances are just one of many challenges faced by the centre in this modern age. Go back

20 or 30 years and the courses and clientele were very different than they are today. Then, it was all about the secondary school pupil. Two-week adventure courses or geography field trips were the meat of the centre's business; St Michaels, Manor, Menzies, Dartmouth, Wodensborough, Churchfields, Alexandra, Wood Green, Stuart Bathurst, George Salter to name but a few. These were all schools that enabled young people to access the benefits of outdoor learning year in year out. Some of them still come for shorter courses and the occasional field trip.

However, changes in the National Curriculum and the establishment of National League tables have called time on the freedom for secondary schools to release students from classroom based learning.

Today's centre caters for a much greater number of children in the primary school age range. The challenge lies in ensuring the flexibility to adapt to a greater range of young people from increasingly diverse backgrounds; from within and from outside the education system. The centre also benefits from the opportunities afforded by the digital era. Google searches, Instagram posts and Facebook follows are all vital in the drive to increase and maintain a healthy and active service to support the people of Sandwell. In this way we enjoy the company of young people from London, Leicestershire, Manchester and Nigeria. This last group come to do the International Duke of Edinburgh Award in late winter/ early spring. They are required to camp each night as part of the award and as the average temperature in Nigeria at that time of the year is somewhere around 40 degrees C - you can imagine the complaining.

One particularly special and in many ways magical course that will always stick in the centre's collective consciousness is when the Encompass course came in 2011. The Encompass team are a collection of young people who come together from across the world to look at conflict resolution. The founders of the organisation are Alex and Mandy Braden, whose son Daniel was killed in the Bali bomb attacks of 2002. This particular course saw a collection of young people from Indonesia, America, the UK, Israel and Palestine. Several people from these last two countries had done National Service in their respective armed forces. Albeit guardedly, the course started well and positive relationships were developing.

Then on Tuesday night the National news reported the deaths of several important Palestinian political figures in an Israeli missile strike. The centre next morning was a micro climate of the escalating anger, mistrust and hatred that flared into outright violence on the West Bank and Gaza strip. It became a mirror to events as they unfolded; events that were beyond our control. Emails and phone calls flew back and forth; two factions formed round two different computers to watch two different versions of the news. The barriers that had slowly begun to lower at the start of the course clanged back into place and seemed more insurmountable than ever. The Encompass group leaders did an incredible job of pulling the two groups together to talk and that afternoon we took them out to a nearby gorge for a bit of outdoor therapy. There's nothing like scrambling up a waterfall and getting a good soaking to help people forget everyday life. As they got wetter and the climbing got harder the smiles got wider and the distrust lessened.

When the group left at the end of that week, (to sighs of relief, it must be said), they did so with a shared experience that helped them to see a person on the other side of the fence and not just a nationality. That course will always stand out as a time when theory and reality merged; when the power of the outdoors was instrumental in shaping human relationships.

Education in its broadest sense is and always has been Plas Gwynant's core belief. Not an education obsessed with targets, numbers and statistics but one where deeper concepts such as communication, acceptance, leadership, friendship and support are presented, unwrapped and carefully developed.

The learning starts the moment an arriving group steps off the coach. Frequently towing bags as large (and occasionally larger) than themselves, the babbling mass make their way through the games room, classroom and finally into their allotted bedrooms where the first challenges of the week take place; unpacking bags and sorting out bedding. It is very easy to see the outdoor centre as a collection of exciting activities that teach life lessons using the climbing rope and the canoe. To overlook the residential side of the centre experience is to miss the myriad small lessons that living together in close confines brings.

To step into any bedroom on a Tuesday afternoon can be an amusing and occasionally daunting prospect. Floors disguised by a layer of strewn, grubby clothes and bathrooms a hotchpotch of bottles, tubes, brushes and towels. It is often Wednesday by the time the average young person realises that the magical spirit that follows them around at home is having a well-earned break and that they must do it themselves. Generally speaking, they sort themselves out. A bedroom tidiness competition usually helps. There is one school which even goes so far as to award extra points for the 'concept' bedroom which has inspired Roman-style drapes and artfully placed dead crabs from the local beach.

At some point the question of the Plas Gwynant ghost is raised. Varying from a man in a de-mob suit, strange footsteps above the dining room (probably the pipes) to the ubiquitous white lady. It must be stressed that no-one can definitively confirm the existence of the paranormal at Plas, but it certainly makes for an interesting night walk and occasionally leads to mild hysteria around bed time; not least amongst the visiting staff in room 4.

It is a long-maintained tradition that all students have a job to do during their stay. Back in the early days this would have involved lighting Tilley lamps and getting the beans on for breakfast. These days we've got them hoovering, laying tables, counting out the recycling and tidying the drying room. The morning jobs are an integral part of the ethos of responsibility that we try to instil. The students are considered part of a family; a unit of people that cares for and has ownership of Plas Gwynant. We often stress the need to 'give back' to the environment that provides their wealth of experience. In doing so, we hope to foster a keen sense of shared respect and ownership for the centre and for each other.

Ultimately, this centre is simply bricks and blocks, quarried out and mortared into shape. What makes it a magic place are the young people who arrive here on a Monday wide eyed, worried and excited. By Friday they are as familiar with Plas, its staff and each other as they are with the street outside their house. They come as strangers and leave as family to the thousands of minds, young and old, whose distant shouts and laughter echo in the corridors down the long years since 1957. Maybe that's the Plas Gwynant ghost. Not a lost spectre wandering the halls but the spirit of a thousand, thousand adventures had since the doors first opened. Ensnared and multiplied with each passing year.

Plas Gwynant has a strong tradition of grass roots outdoor adventure and the modern centre has maintained that proud tradition. In the last 20 years the outdoor industry has taken off in a way that few could really have foreseen. Type 'Outdoor Adventure' into a search engine and you'll come up with hundreds of colourful and highly attractive opportunities to slide on zip lines, scramble round ropes courses, jump from cranes and planes, Zorb across lakes (you'll have to find out for yourself), throw yourself into the sea and climb virtually anything imaginable.

The methods of interacting with the outdoor environment are seemingly endless and there are more and more people getting into 'Adventure'.

Plas has always been about immersing young people in the natural environment using activities that provide lifelong lessons. Today's pre-course liaison process requires group leaders to focus carefully on what they want to achieve with their young people as opposed to asking what activities they want to do. This strong ethos of putting the individual before the activity has been the centre's core belief for a long time. Phil Watkin was an instructor at the centre between 1974 and 1994. As a young graduate of the Bangor University teacher training programme, Phil was looking for an outdoor position that spoke to his beliefs on the development of young people. After several visits to similar centres he came to an interview at Plas Gwynant and immediately connected with what he found. "We're into putting the kids first here," said the then deputy head of centre, peering over his glasses in a meaningful way. 20 years later Phil only retired as his knees were giving him grief.

So, what does 'kids first' actually mean? Well, one way of structuring a weekly programme is to base it around the activity. Tuesday climb, Wednesday canoe, Thursday up a mountain etc. The programme is established on a Monday and there is no variation except for fire, flood and natural disaster. There are merits to this as instructors can organise logistics in advance. But what if it becomes apparent that a group of students allotted to a particular instructor struggle with their communication skills and argue like cat and dog? What if their physical ability and confidence is low and they need to start the week with an activity that bonds them together and teaches them to look each other in the eye, stretch out a hand and give each other a bunk up? To open the week with a climbing session that requires patience, trust and communication could well be setting them up to fail. A group like that would be better suited to scrambling up a mountain gorge. The inherent group challenge and fluidity of waterfall climbing is an ideal way to open young minds to the need to be a strong team. Suddenly they're up and running and they start to understand. Their minds envelop a set of ideas that suddenly mean something. They realise that if they don't support each other and communicate effectively then they won't succeed.

So now a switch has been thrown, the challenge is in maintaining momentum?

The objectives for the week could be to develop the group's ability to see the strengths inherent in the entire team and they're also studying mountains and rivers at school, so a day exploring the hills above Beddgelert would be perfect. There's a lovely ridgeline that sweeps up from the bottom of the Glaslyn gorge, which offers tricky but attainable climbing and breath-taking views over the foothills and floodplains stretching towards Porthmadog. An ideal opportunity to combine challenge, encouragement and a vision of the meeting of the mountains and the sea. By the end of the day they're footsore and tired. What better way forward is there than a day canoeing and maybe some focussed team challenges on the rocks by the coast. There's nothing quite like canoeing to hammer home the need to communicate effectively. As the boat gently spins across the lake and is lodged in the trees… yet again… to the backdrop of raised, bickering voices, it is easy to wonder if they've listened to a word that's been said all week! Then suddenly someone remembers that day in the gorge; how they listened to each other and had a leader who pulled together the ideas and came up with a plan. Lo and behold, the boat gently backs out of the bushes, turns and heads off in something resembling a straight line. Six paddles dip in and out of the lake in shaky unison and most importantly, six minds understand the need to act as one if they are going to achieve success.

The wonderful thing about being tucked away in the middle of Snowdonia National park is that it provides the opportunities to create adventures for people of all ages. A mountain day can be a low-level woodland walk with some den building, hide and seek and tree identification. It can also be a complex and difficult ridgeline sweeping up the flanks of Snowdon to deposit you above the cloud on the highest mountain top in Wales and England. A canoe or kayak session can be a placid lake journey to a remote spot for a campfire and marshmallows. It can also be teaching the skills to successfully run rapids or surf an ocean wave. There are gorges that require waterfall leaps and scary climbs and there are ones in which it is possible to give a group of 11year olds the tools to look after themselves.

There are days when we don helmet and head torch and worm our way into the subterranean world beneath the mountains, to explore the passages and caverns of abandoned slate mines. Some groups hire mountain bikes and learn the skills necessary to go off road and some come to point a camera and gain a GCSE in creativity. The opportunities for alternative adventures are as diverse as the groups who come but the common threads of enjoyment, fun, life experience and learning run through all.

It is said that the proof of the pudding is in the eating. A fitting proverb for the centre's work as students regularly provides insights that prove the worth of the experience. Very few weeks go by without someone saying something that we've not heard before. There will be a spin or variation in understanding of leadership, communication, recognition of the strengths inherent in all of us, the need to be positive and accept mistakes, trust, respect, friendship.... the list goes on.

Conservation and environmental awareness have also become an increasing part of the life of the centre. Several years ago, Plas attained the National Eco-Centre status in recognition of the work it does in relation to developing environmental awareness among young people. The scheme is no longer in operation nationwide, but the centre has taken ownership of the concepts. In addition to everyday recycling, energy conservation and waste reduction some groups take part in active conservation projects as part of the John Muir Award scheme. This is a nationally recognised award that combines adventure and exploration with an active 'giving back' task. Bashing bracken around tree plantations and ripping up invasive rhododendrons to allow native species to flourish is always popular. There's nothing like a bit of sanctioned destruction to keep the interest up. Some groups have also been involved in a community project in Beddgelert, the local village, to rejuvenate the community garden. This work is being done in partnership with local residents and National Park wardens. Young people from Sandwell are taking responsibility for their environment and developing their understanding of communities different to their own.

So, what does the future hold for Plas Gwynant Outdoor education centre?

Wouldn't it be wonderful to have the benefit of a crystal ball allowing access to the future? Something that would allow plans to be laid with the benefit of concrete knowledge. In the absence of such a tool adaptability is the key to survival, just as it is when out walking on the hills. The winds of fortune bring changing weather and circumstance. A centre that can flex and adapt is one that gives itself the greatest chance of success. Plas Gwynant's future can draw from the strength in its past.

Back in May 2017 we hosted the yearly re-union weekend for slightly more mature students to get together and play in the outdoors. The majority of the participants first came to the centre in the 1960s on month-long or two-week courses. The weather that May weekend was glorious, particularly on Saturday. Sunny spells all day, early spring warmth and a gentle westerly wind. Perfect for a canoe expedition on the Menai Straits; the body of water that separates main land Wales from Anglesey. The tides were perfect for a west to east trip from Felinheli to Menai Bridge. The sky was a little greyer than we would have liked when we put-on in our rafted canoes. As we swung onto the magic carpet of the pushing tide the sun broke free and picked out the distant Britannia and Menai Bridges and the nearby bulk of Plas Newydd, the Marquis of Anglesey's mansion. We had our lunch gently drifting on the tide and breeze and then readied ourselves for the strong tidal streams that rush though the stanchions of the first of the yawning bridges.

Whipping through at pace we dropped behind the old fish smokehouse to rest in a back eddy. Looking around at the group, everyone wore a smile as wide as a mile. Every face flushed and breathless as the excitement, the beauty of the place, the tang in the air and the building rush of the water infected us equally.

In that moment was caught a tangible glimpse of the power of outdoor education and the long-term impact Plas Gwynant had on a group of individuals. However, there was one member in particular who encapsulated the scope and spread of it all. I'm sure he won't mind his name being mentioned here.

Wally Gough, who occupied the front of one of the boats and who was probably getting splashed the most, first came to the centre in 1958, the year it opened as an adventure school. Here he was, 60 years on, paddle in hand, out there having a go and still loving the buzz of the adventure - laughing aloud at life. In that moment of captured glee, the sense of history was as tangible as the sea.

How many more lives have been touched in this way over the years? How many more memories are there of sunny days on mountain tops, teetering around on rock faces, being dunked in cold lakes, companionship and challenge, success and lessons learned? Who knows? But like one of the many great trees towering in the centre grounds, planted when the house was first built, each new experience is a fresh branch, twig or leaf sprouting from the strong limbs of adventures past.

And so, with each passing season, grows the whole.

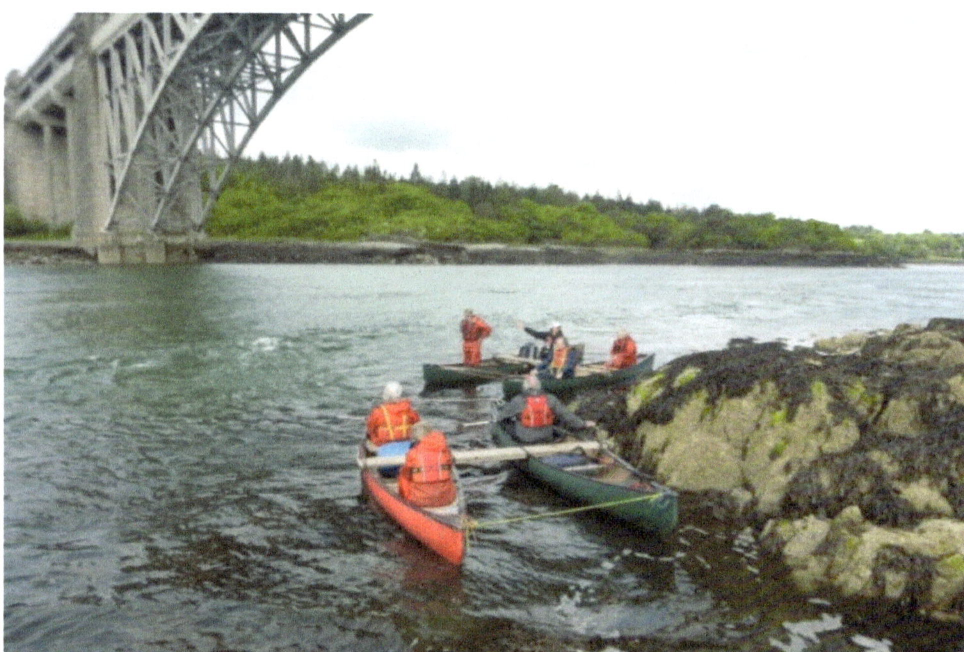

Kevin Bird, Tutor

What Plas Gwynant means to me...

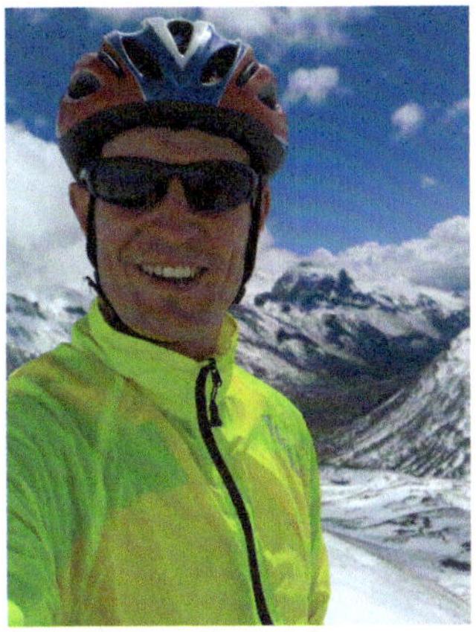

I started my time at Plas just before the new millennium began, thinking it was just another short term contract in an otherwise 'bitty' outdoor career. Eighteen years later and I'm still here and still marvelling at what the young (and not so young!) people achieve when they come here. The comments we get range from: "This is the best week of my life" to "This place is sick!" to "You're the best tour guide ever!" To be honest, I was a little disappointed at the last comment, wondering whether I was perhaps missing something in the way I had been teaching the students... I'm sure there was just a little lost in translation as they say!

During my time here there have been a lot of changes: changes in staff, in management, in the type of courses we offer, in the activities we do...the list goes on. But the one thing that has remained a constant throughout is the overall ethos of the centre to provide high quality residential outdoor education to young people. And the young people keep coming, supported by incredible staff, and keep on achieving things they never thought possible. And that's why I'm still here, and hopefully will be for many years to come.

Mladenka (Mel) Hooper, Tutor

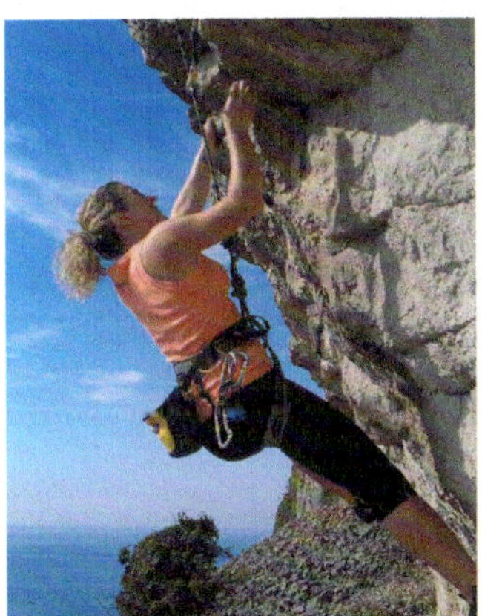

In terms of period that this book will cover and also compared to the length of time some staff been working in Plas Gwynant, I am relative newbie. I've been working in the centre for three full years now, but it seems like only yesterday that I started. I have enjoyed every moment of it and despite originally having plans to go abroad, work and travel after a few years in Plas, I have a feeling that I will be working here until I retire! I just love working in Plas, it is the perfect working environment. Perfect location, beautiful grounds and buildings, great values and ethics and a very strong, well bonded brilliant team from management to kitchen staff.

There is always a great relaxed atmosphere and I find it very easy to get on with everyone. Even in the short time I've been here I've witnessed how Plas is changing and adapting to new challenges. It manages to keep up with the changing times but its core values and magic touch is ever present. Working with both the kids and adults is rewarding as you can see how the experiences not only develop them but also give them a better insight into their own abilities and potential. To see the positive changes in the individuals during their short residential here is both rewarding and joyful for myself.

Dominic Roe
A year (and a bit!) as a Centre Assistant

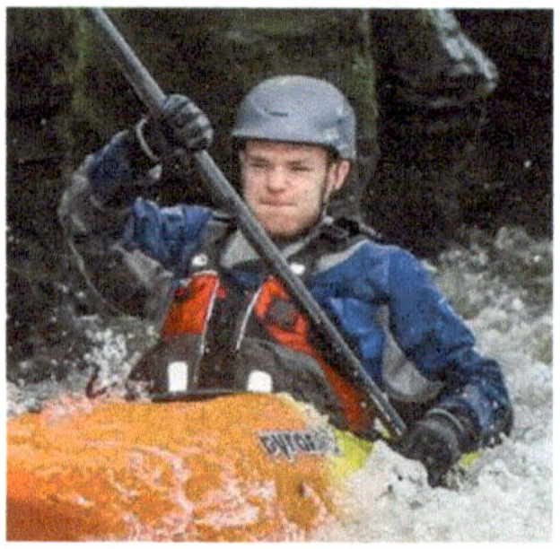

I joined the team at Plas Gwynant in June 2016, having finished a three-year teaching degree and deciding that teaching in the classroom was not my cup of tea.

I thought of different ways I could continue to teach young-people new skills and being a keen climber and mountain biker, with a background in mountaineering, I thought outdoor education was worth a look! The centre assistant scheme has been a brilliant way of getting into the profession. I started off working with groups a couple of days a week as an assistant instructor, before being allowed to run more and more of the week independently, as I became more competent.

This year has been a great way to learn from the wealth of knowledge that we're lucky to have at Plas, as well as meet the wide variety of schools and staff we get through the doors!
I'm fortunate enough to have been given the opportunity to complete my summer Mountain Leader award, as well as the training aspect of my SPA (climbing) and gained really useful skills in leading every activity that Plas offer. Being able to work with such a wide range of students throughout the year has taught me far more than you can ever get from a textbook.

Unfortunately, the centre assistant scheme was only a year-long and my time at Plas came to an end in August. Having accepted a trainee position at a much larger centre in North Yorkshire, I'm looking forward to the new experiences that lie ahead and the skills, friends and life that comes with it. I hope the next centre assistant will enjoy their time here just as much as I have!

Best bits - The homemade cakes and biscuits.
Worst bits - Sweeping out the stores on a Friday!
What I'll miss the most - Having Snowdonia on my doorstep.
(From the Plas Gwynant Newsletter Dated June 2017)

Deb Hughes
Former Administrator at Plas Gwynant 27 April 1998 – 18 November 2016

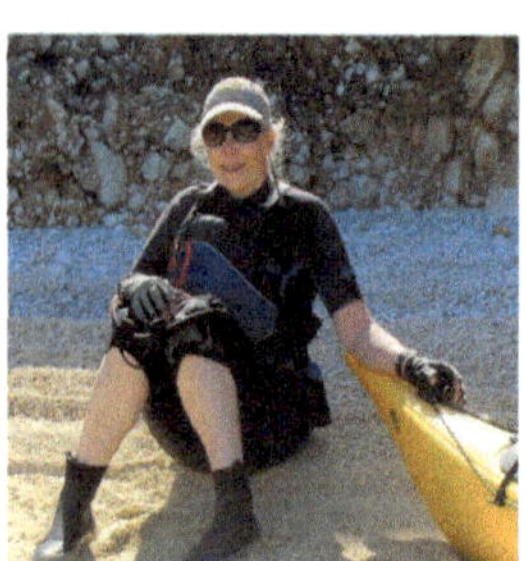

I started working as Administrator at Plas Gwynant in April 1998. I had no idea then the impact working at the centre would have on my life. I knew nothing about the outdoor world when I went there. Schools came and went and I had little contact with them.

As time went on I became more curious about what they got up to on a visit and through staff training days began to become more involved with what went on outside the office. Two week courses for secondary schools were the norm throughout the summer term, focussing on PSE and adventure, giving much more time for the tutors to challenge students and bring out the best in their groups. At the end of the course the students were given a report card and certificate which listed all the activities they had undertaken during the week. Ascent of Tryfan, Snowdon, Moel Siabod, kayaking at Black Rock Sands, Canoeing on Llyn Gwynant etc., I was responsible for typing these certificates up and can remember asking what is the difference between kayaking and canoeing? That was the beginning of a very long journey into the realms of kayaking which has led to amazing paddling trips in a variety of far flung places.

There have been many challenges along the way and some scary bits, but no regrets. I would never have had the courage to do half the stuff I have done were it not for the ethos of Plas Gwynant and can see that even short visits to the centre of 5 days or so has had an amazing effect on many, many of Sandwell's students.

This began to dawn on me as while working in the office, I would often see people wandering about the grounds and I would go and check what they were up to. They turned out to be people who had been to Plas Gwynant with their schools, some of them a very long time ago, who wanted to come back and see if the place was still the same. They were all thrilled to be back and recounted tales of their exploits whilst here.

The overwhelming impression that came over from these returnees was that their visit to Plas was the best thing that had happened to them whilst at school and the thing they remembered most. I began to take contact details from people and eventually had a very long list. The idea of a Plas Gwynant Reunion was born and although we missed the 50th anniversary of the opening of the centre by a year or so, a very enthusiastic gang of former students arrived for a weekend of activities and socialising in May 2010(?) There were students who came on the very first three week pilot course in 1958 and some from the 60s and 70s, all thrilled to be back at Plas Gwynant to relive their exploits. The reunion weekends became an annual event by popular demand and have gone from strength to strength. With only one lady on the first weekend, more ladies have since joined in the fun.

It is sad to see other LEA centres in North Wales closing due to budget pressures and the problems schools have in releasing students from curriculum demands etc., but I feel it is one of those 'you don't know what you've got till it's gone' situations.

Plas Gwynant has had a tremendous effect on so many young people's lives, giving the students of Sandwell such a wonderful chance to experience so many things - besides the obvious outdoor activities - being away from home, the social aspect of living with their fellow students, the spiritual experience of being out in the wild world without the trappings of their everyday lives back in Sandwell.

The Centre is a treasure – here's to the next 60 years!

Last, but by no means least, the Plas Gwynant Cooks!

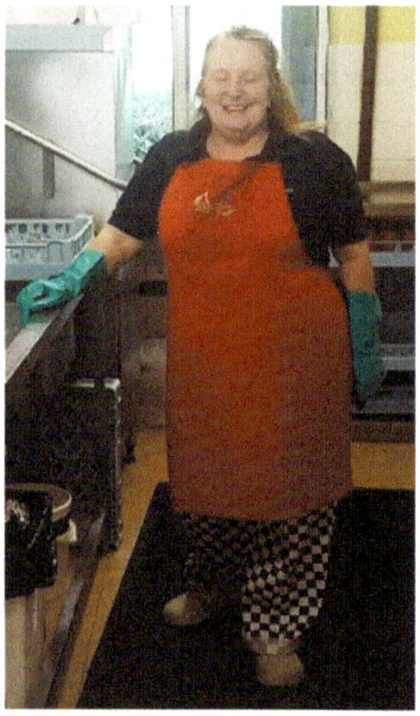

There is no doubt that the meals produced by the renowned cooks at Plas Gwynant are a key factor in providing the lifelong memories of Plas Gwynant.

To fully appreciate the adventures, it is imperative to start the day with a hearty breakfast. By the same token it is good to tuck into the evening meal after a full days' activity in Snowdonia.

Wendy and Janice are today's cooks, providing sustenance to all intrepid visitors at Plas.

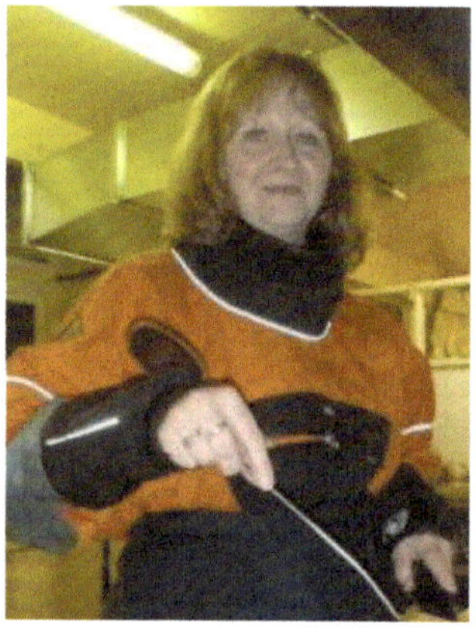

Hats off to the culinary skills of the Plas Gwynant cooks, past and present!

Extracts from the Plas Gwynant Website

At Plas Gwynant we believe having the right staff team is our biggest asset. All staff at Plas Gwynant enjoy working with young people and work hard to create a welcoming family feel to the place. We strive to make sure every visitor feels valued and secure within an environment that encourages them to reach their potential. We understand that a residential course extends beyond activities and ensure that support staff and tutorial staff are fully involved with resident groups to give them the best experience we can. Whether it's climbing a mountain, keeping the centre clean, cooking meals, managing the grounds or the liaison process we will always seek to be as supportive as possible and do the best we can. Our tutorial staff team brings a breadth of professional experience and qualifications in delivering outdoor education and activity courses to young people from a wide variety of age groups and backgrounds. The tutorial staff and support staff can often be found on mountains, rivers, lakes and the sea when not at work and are up to date with the skills, knowledge and practice required to deliver safe educational experiences within adventurous settings.

Plas Gwynant offers a wide range of high quality adventurous outdoor activities suitable from the age of 10 upwards that make the best use of the surrounding environment. We are lucky to be located in a stunning part of Snowdonia National Park, just North of Beddgelert in North Wales, where we have easy access to mountains, cliffs, lakes, rivers, gorges, forests, beaches and the sea often within walking distance or a short minibus journey. Activities include: Mountain Walking,

Rock Climbing, Abseiling, Gorge Walking, Sea Level Traversing, Canoeing, Kayaking, Raft Building, Beach Exploration, Mine Exploration, Environmental Based Activities, Orienteering, Problem Solving, Bush Craft and Mountain Biking. Courses provided for: Primary Schools, Secondary Schools, Further and Higher Education, INSET and Teacher Courses, Youth Groups, Adult Courses, Holiday Courses, Corporate Training and John Muir Award. Availability of courses are displayed on the website.

We are able to cater for a wide variety of groups up to a maximum size of 48 plus 6 staff.
New facilities mean that groups do not have to commit to the whole centre and that the centre is also available for groups of 30 students, plus up to 4 staff or 20 students plus 2 staff. Groups can either choose to work together or be independent. We provide a welcoming and personal approach to learning. Plas Gwynant offers unique outdoor experiences within a beautiful and inspirational setting.

In a recent survey of 37 schools and groups that have used us in the last year 79% rated the value of the experience as outstanding with the remaining 21% rating us as good.

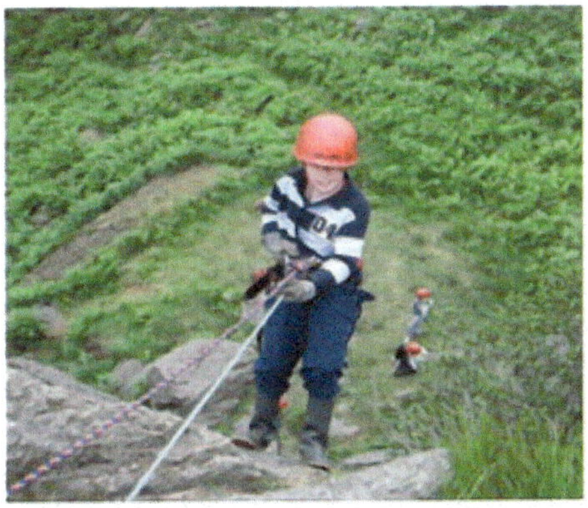

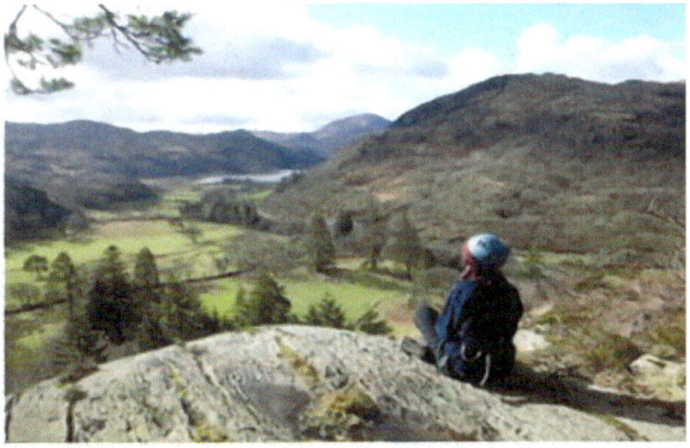

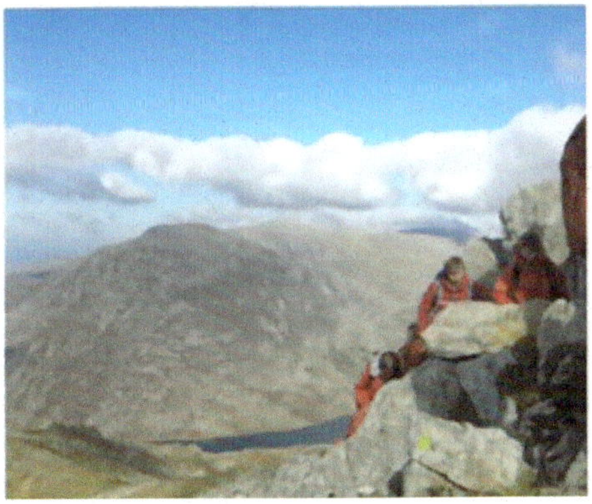

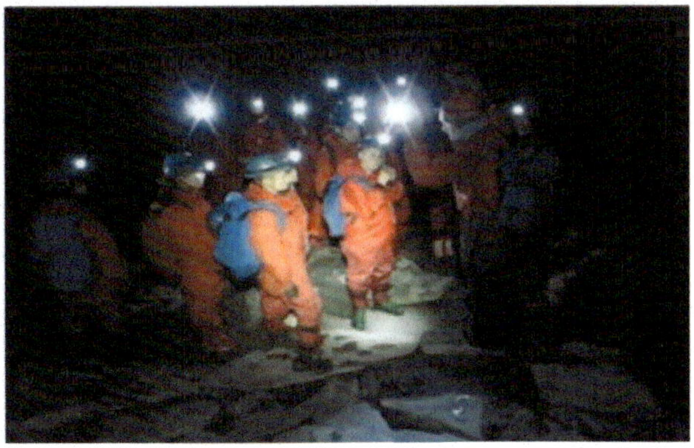

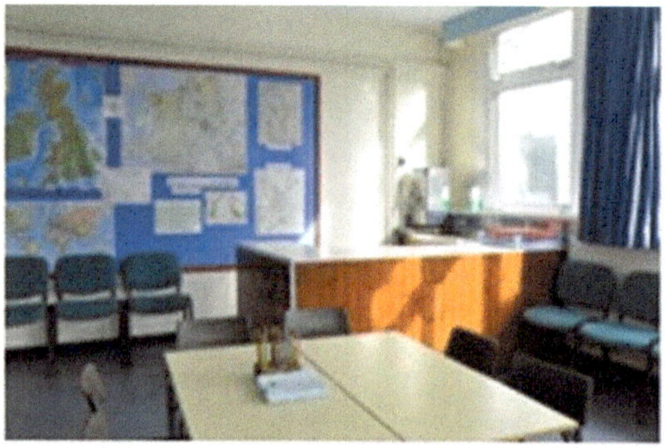
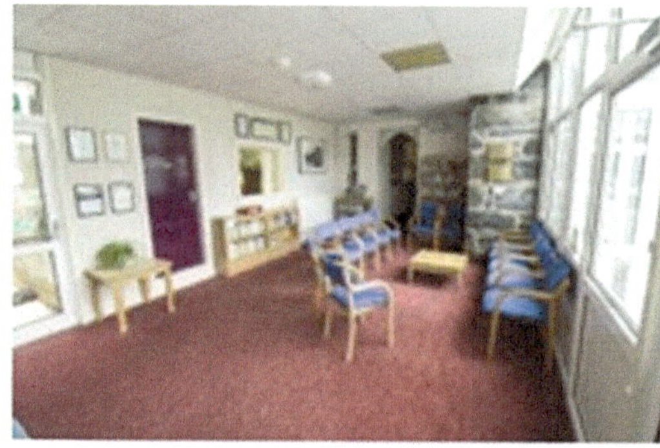
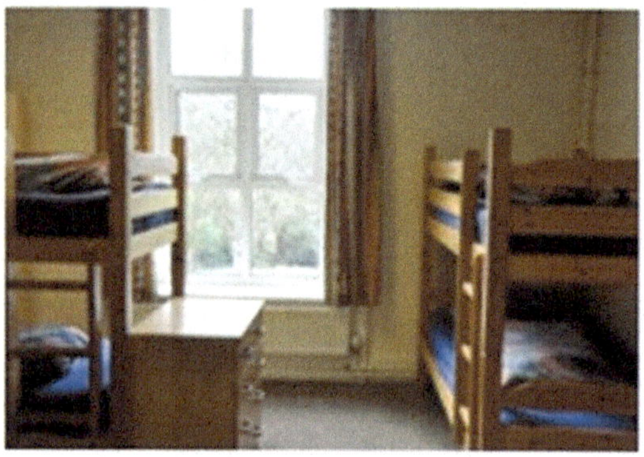
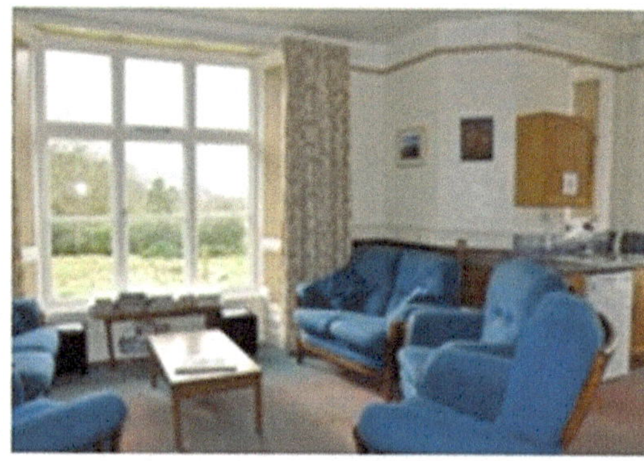
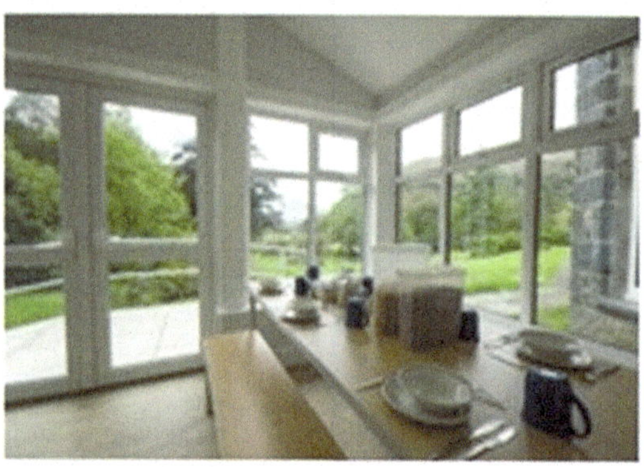
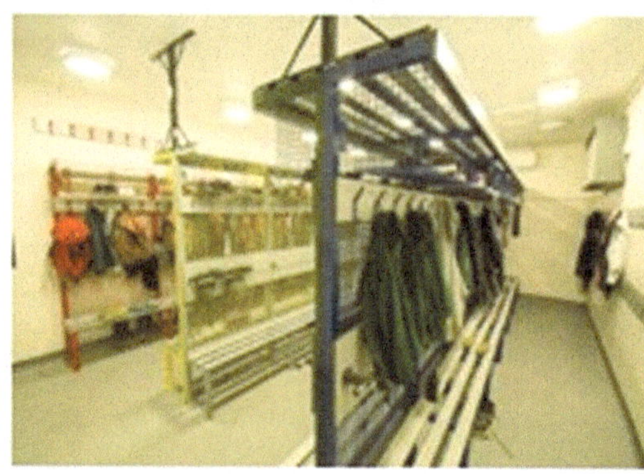
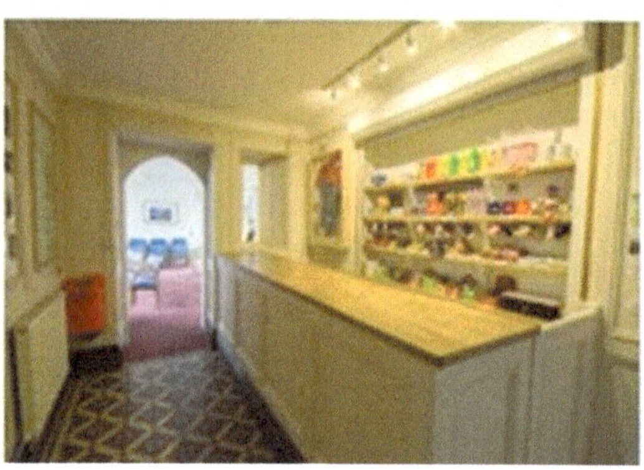
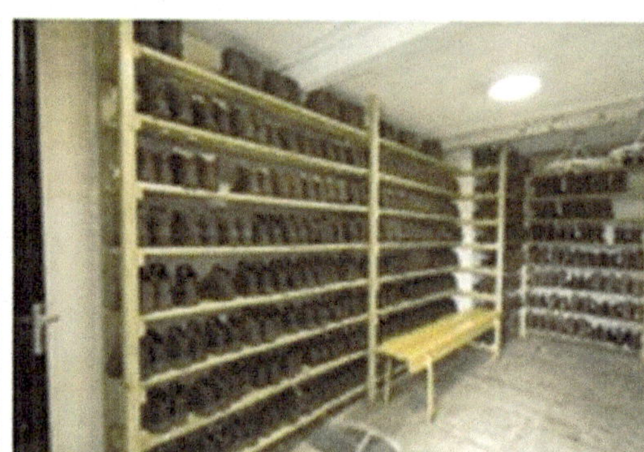

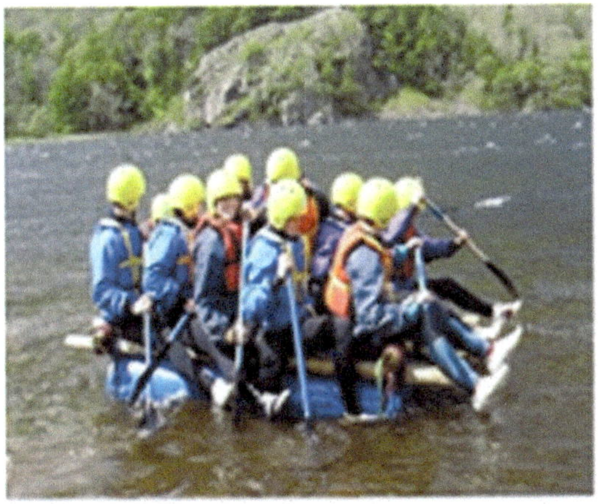

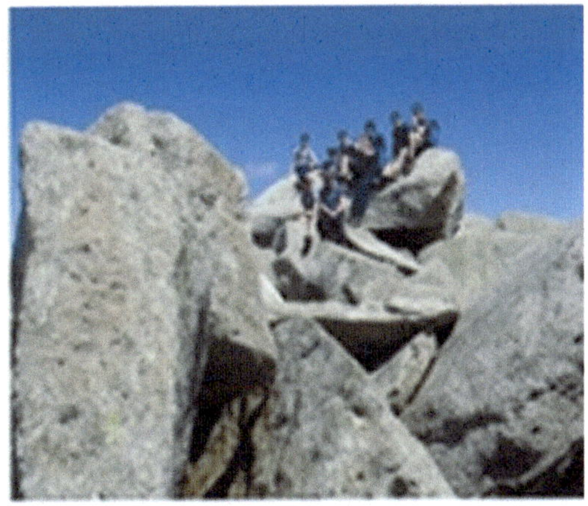

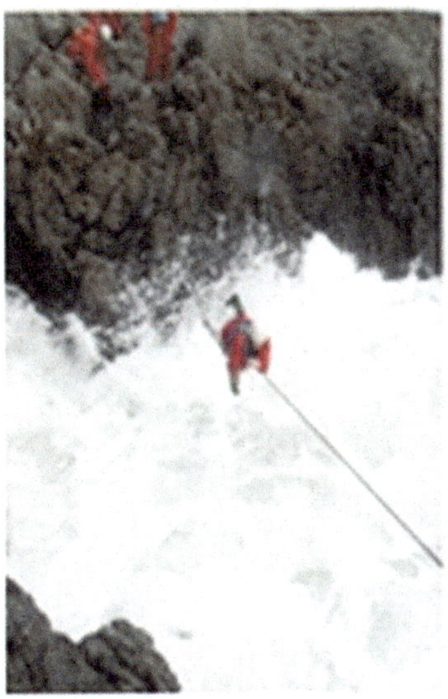

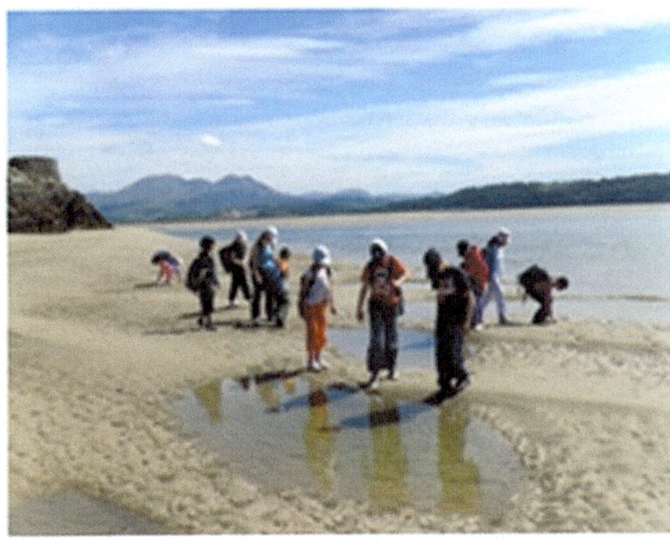

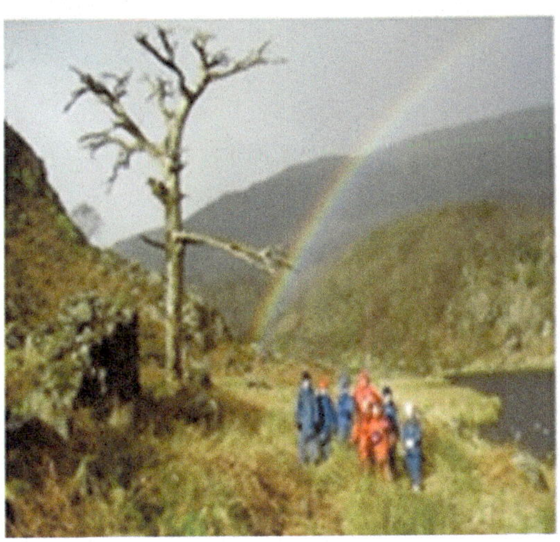

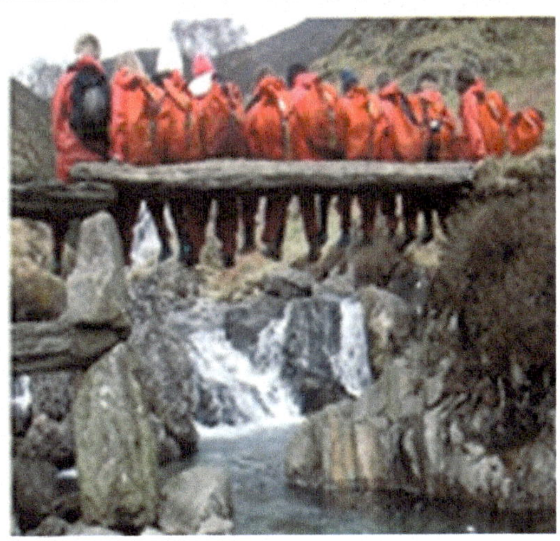

~ ACKNOWLEDGEMENTS ~

This celebratory book would not have been possible without the wonderful memories and photographs shared by so many people, whose passion for Plas Gwynant has not diminished over the years.

The mountaineering club of the early 1950s whose members included Bert Wright, Physical Education Adviser at West Bromwich Council, who passed on the idea of purchasing a run-down property to Mr Turner, the Director of Education, who in turn supported the idea and influenced council members to approve the purchase. And the early instructors who pioneered the outward bound ethos and helped formulate the success of courses at Plas Gwynant, which would benefit thousands of students throughout the decades that followed, (some still coming to annual reunion weekends more than half a century later and enjoying activities as they once had as schoolchildren).

Testament to the success of the venture is documented here for posterity and our grateful thanks go to the many contributors, each sharing their experience of Plas Gwynant through the decades, and to the present staff, Richard Oakes, Jeff Handley, Dan Jackson, Kevin Bird, Mel Hooper, et al, whose vision for the future is just as exciting as the original concept.

In recognition of all contributors, duly noted (in alphabetical order) –

Olwyn Bailey
Roger Bainbridge
Patrick Belshaw
Kevin Bird
Sir Chris Bonington CBE
Steven Edwards
June Fletcher
Roger (Paul) Freeman
Wally Gough
William Hall
Jeff Handley
Eddie Hannington
Mladenka (Mel) Hooper
Debbie Hughes
Dan Jackson
Ken Latham
Derrick Lees

Chris Martin
John Murden
Richard Oakes
Brenda Murtha
Michael Page
Derek Poulton
Dominic Roe
Gary Rushton
Roy Simms
Reg Snell
Geoffrey Turner
John Turton
Pat Turton
Murray Watterson OBE
Peter Wharton
Rosemary Winnall MBE
Lynn Woodward
Bert Wright

With special thanks to Lisa Simone Jones for her amazing help.

~ REFERENCES ~

The New Naturalist: *'Snowdon: The National Park of North Wales'* by F J North, Bruce Campbell and Richenda Scott, 1949

Several extracts from the pamphlet produced by John Murden for Sandwell Department of Education *'Plas Gwynant: The First 25 Years 1958-1983'*.

Llyn Gwynant - From *'The Lakes of Eryri'* by Geraint Roberts

Ghost Stories from Plas Gwynant - Extracts from *'Bedd Gelert its Facts, Fairies & Folklore'* 1899 by D E Jenkins, Porthmadog, Editor of *'Cyfres Ieuenctid Cymru'*

Extract from *'The Cronehillians'* School Magazine 1959 - First Pilot Course 1958. Contribution from pupils Nick Tarr, D Wall, J Morris, Form 5 – West Bromwich Secondary Technical School

Extract from *'Forever Churchfields'* book, Contribution from Fred Luke - PE Teacher at Churchfields High School

Extract from E G Rowland's publication *'Hill Walking in Snowdonia'* regarding the Brocken Spectre.

Extracts from *'West Bromwich Mountaineering Club: The first 50 years'* by founder members - Bert Wright, Geoff Robinson, Ted Hutton, Martin Bessell, Hughie Young, Rev Keith Treacher, Peter Woodward, Ray Vaughan, Mike Thompson and Wally Cheeseborough. (With kind permission from David Jones, Committee Chair)

http://footlesscrow.blogspot.co.uk/2014/01/the-scottie-how-first-climbing-nut-was.html

http://plasgwynant.org.uk/

http://www.beddgelerttourism.com

Sandwell CHAS (Sandwell Community History and Archives Service)